ASK THE DOCTOR ABOUT
PARKINSON'S DISEASE

Ask the Doctor About Parkinson's Disease

MICHAEL S. OKUN, MD

HUBERT H. FERNANDEZ, MD

demos
HEALTH
New York

Visit our website at www.demosmedpub.com

LIBRARY OF CONGRESS CATALOGING-IN-PUBLICATION DATA
. . . .
Okun, Michael S.
    Ask the doctor about Parkinson's disease / Michael S. Okun, Hubert H. Fernandez.
    p. cm.
Includes bibliographical references and index.
ISBN 978–1–932603–81–1 (alk. paper)
1. Parkinson's disease—Miscellanea. I. Fernandez, Hubert H. II. Title.
RC382.O474 2010
616.8'33—dc22   2009024709

Special discounts on bulk quantities of Demos Health books
are available to corporations, professional associations, pharmaceutical companies, health care
organizations, and other qualifying groups. For details, please contact:

Special Sales Department
Demos Medical Publishing
11 W. 42nd Street, 15th Floor
New York, NY 10036
Phone: 800–532–8663 or 212–683–0072
Fax: 212–941–7842
Email: rsantana@demosmedpub.com

Made in the United States of America
09   10   11   12   13   5   4   3   2   1

This book is dedicated to the National Parkinson Foundation and their tireless efforts to help Parkinson's disease patients and families. All royalties from the book will be donated to the National Parkinson Foundation.

Contents

Preface   ix

1. Parkinson's Disease: What Is It?   3
2. Adjusting to Life With Parkinson's Disease   43
3. Motor Symptoms   61
4. Nonmotor Symptoms   75
5. Pharmacological Approaches to Treatment   97
6. Alternative and Complementary Approaches
    to Treatment   131
7. Multidisciplinary Approaches to Treatment   151
8. Surgical Approaches to Treatment   167
9. Stem Cells, Gene Therapy, Transplants, and
    Other Medical Treatments   191
10. Ten Things on the Horizon for Treating
    Parkinson's Disease   205

Appendix   207
Resources   215
Further Reading   221
About the Authors   223
Index   227

Preface

One of the greatest honors of our lives has been to serve as physicians, researchers, teachers, confidants, and as friends to Parkinson's disease patients and their families. The truth is, we have learned much more from you than we could ever hope to pay back. We write this book for you, who have deeply inspired and moved us, and we hope that in some small way this can repay a debt of gratitude. You have enriched our lives and made us better people. We have had the privilege of moderating the free web-based question and answer section of the Ask the Doctor forum at the National Parkinson Foundation (www.parkinson.org) for the last three years, and we have had the chance to answer thousands of questions and interact with amazing numbers of patients and families. Questions have been received and answered from six continents (not Antarctica yet). We realize that many of you have no access to medical care or access to specialized Parkinson's care, and we pray that we have been able to provide you with the guidance necessary to enhance the quality of your lives.

We have had the privilege of traveling the world to promote Parkinson's disease awareness, and, in addition to the website, we have had the opportunity to travel with you, see how you live, and answer your questions in lectures and in town hall forum formats. We therefore have been able to draw from our interactions with you on the website, your in-person questions, and from articles we have penned for the foundation (the *Parkinson Report* and the "What's Hot" website column). Additionally, we have worked as Parkinson's disease and movement disorders scientists and together have penned hundreds of articles on relevant topics including everything from cutting edge research to education and outreach.

In this book we aim to bring all of these experiences together in a comprehensive question-and-answer format. When writing the book we found that we had so many excellent questions from patients and caregivers that we decided to include an extra 15 questions and answers in order to be as complete as possible. The scenarios we describe and discuss are from real life, however we have taken the liberty of expanding the details of the dialogue. We have also provided recent reference articles and books.

We have enjoyed working on this project immensely, and we hope that the content will help and inspire you. In these difficult economic times, we will continue to raise money to support the amazing science of care delivery programs and the centers of excellence offered by the National Parkinson Foundation. We will be donating the royalties of this book to the National Parkinson Foundation, so by purchasing a copy of this book you are helping the Parkinson's disease cause. If you would like to make further contributions or to place the National Parkinson Foundation on your list of yearly charitable contributions, we could think of no better way to honor you than to put your money to work combating this challenging disease.

To make a gift by mail: National Parkinson Foundation, Inc., Office of Development, 1501 NW 9th Avenue/Bob Hope Road, Miami, Florida, 33136-1494

To make a gift by phone: 1-800-327-4545 (toll-free in the U.S.)

To make a gift online: www.parkinson.org

Michael S. Okun
Hubert H. Fernandez

ASK THE DOCTOR ABOUT PARKINSON'S DISEASE

I was diagnosed with Parkinson's disease about 2 months ago (I'm 45, female, and in very good health otherwise). My dad was diagnosed with Parkinson's disease about 11 years ago and he is still self-sufficient. My paternal grandparents had neurological problems and because there were limited diagnostic capabilities at the time (they lived in Italy) and even less understanding of Parkinson's disease, I'm not sure whether they had the disease ... but my grandmother had tremors and my grandfather had other neurological disorders.

Given my history, I'm wondering if I may have the form of Parkinson's disease that is caused by genetic mutation. If so, is there any way for me to test for that genetic mutation at this time?

CHAPTER 1

Parkinson's Disease: What Is It?

What are the symptoms that may be clues to the onset of Parkinson's disease?

There are many potential symptoms and/or signs that may signal the earliest features and/or evidence supporting a diagnosis of Parkinson's disease (PD). It is estimated that a person must lose approximately 60% (or more) of the dopamine-producing brain cells (referred to as the *substantia nigra*, which means the "black substance" in Latin) before noticeable changes will be detected. This cell loss always occurs before the symptoms that set off suspicion in patients, family members, or even doctors. This situation of a "threshold" of cell loss that must be eclipsed for appearance of symptoms can be compared to what may occur in patients who experience kidney failure. When a kidney begins to malfunction, approximately 75% or more of its cells are lost, and those cells are unrecoverable. Frustratingly for kidney failure patients, the routine laboratory tests are almost always normal and hint abnormality only when the failure process has already begun. In PD, as in kidney failure, a threshold of cells must be lost before symptoms manifest in a person.

Many scientists have turned their attention to searching for presymptomatic (before the diagnosis) screening tests. These tests have been designed to try to detect PD prior to the loss of a large number of these important brain cells. Presymptomatic research has focused on areas such as smell testing (sniffing), cognitive screening (tests of thinking), imaging (magnetic resonance imaging [MRI] and other advanced brain pictures), and blood markers (things that can be detected in the blood like a sugar or glucose level). Currently there is no reliable biomarker for PD, with the

exception of a small number of families who carry known genetic mutations (changes in their DNA) for the disease.

Sometimes the symptoms of PD can be very obvious, such as a resting tremor. In many instances, however, they are subtle and may manifest in ways a general doctor may not immediately identify with PD (eg,
smaller than normal handwriting [micrographia], shoulder pain, or a
decreased arm swing). The easiest symptoms to detect are considered to
be the common motor symptoms, and these usually occur more promi-
nently on one side of the body. The reason why PD is worse on one side
of the body as compared to the other (asymmetric symptoms) remains
a mystery.

The common motor symptoms of PD may include (a) tremor (shakiness), (b) stiffness (rigidity), (c) slowness (bradykinesia), (d) soft voice
(hypophonia), (e) shuffling steps (and the shuffling steps may be accompanied by festination, or chasing the center of gravity with short steps—
the patient may appear to be tripping in a forward direction), (f) freezing,
balance problems, (g) start hesitation, (h) micrographia, or (i) loss of facial
expression (masked face).

It is important to keep in mind that 20% of patients will not have resting tremor and also that a small number of patients may present initially
with depression or sleep disorders (1–8).

When does PD really start?

This is one of the million dollar questions in PD research. We actually do
not know the answer. From the clinical trial or research perspective, we
arbitrarily base the answer on either the occurrence of the first symptom
or alternatively the date of diagnosis (but we do not really know). The
date of diagnosis is, however, biased and largely based on obvious motor
symptoms such as tremor, stiffness, or slowness. We know that this esti-
mate therefore is grossly inaccurate. In fact, by the time a person with
Parkinson's (PWP) manifests the first symptom (eg, tremor of the fingers),
significant degeneration (ie, loss of brain cells) of the dopaminergic neurons in the brain has already occurred.

We now know that the loss of the sense of smell, constipation, depression, personality changes, sleep problems, and even anxiety may long precede the motor symptoms of PD. The problem with using these symptoms
as diagnostic markers, however, is that they commonly occur in the general population, making it very difficult to judge what is part of PD and
what is not (9–11).

Complicating the picture as to the onset of PD has been the discovery
that many patients may have rapid eye movement (REM) sleep disorders

(ie, when patients attempt to act out their dreams) many years prior to the onset of motor symptoms (12–15). In addition, Braak and colleagues have recently proposed that the degeneration in PD actually starts well before dopaminergic cells in the midbrain begin to die (16–21).

What is the history of PD?

PD, sometimes erroneously termed *paralysis agitans*, was described in the Indian medical system of Ayurveda (called Kampavata) and also by Galen (AD 175) who referred to it as the shaking palsy. Perhaps the most interesting reference came from Shakespeare, who wrote in Henry VI "why dost thou quiver man?" The character in the story responds by saying "the palsy and not the fear provokes me." The use of the term Parkinson's was largely credited to the highly influential 19th-century French neurologist Jean-Martin Charcot, although it should be noted that many people prior to Parkinson himself described the disease. James Parkinson (1755–1824), a Londoner and son of an apothecary and surgeon, is credited with the eponym for his 1817 essay on the shaking palsy. His descriptions included six cases of which only three were actually examined (of the other three, two were met on the street and one simply observed) (22–36).

What is the history of the discovery of levodopa?

There were several seminal discoveries that led to the development of levodopa as a therapy for PD.

1911—First synthesis of its D,L racemate and the isolation of its L-isomer from the seedling of Vicia faba beans

1913—Isolation from legumes (pea plant family)

1930—L-dopa was shown to have an effect on rabbit glucose metabolism

1938—L-dopa decarboxylase described and enzymatic conversion to dopamine demonstrated

1940—Studies on the effects of L-dopa on blood vessels

1950—Studies began to consider the use of dopamine on the brain

1960–1961—Consideration was given to PD treatment, which was found to be related to dopamine (throughout the 1960s there were inconsistent responses to treatment)

1967—High-dose levodopa was verified for treatment of PWPs (Dr. George Cotzias)

1970s—Dopamine decarboxylase was added to the regimen to improve the side effect profile and absorption.

Many scientists have worked on the development of levodopa and levodopa therapy, and the list of their names is too long for this short book. Arvid Carlsson from Sweden won the Nobel Prize in 2000 for his work on the administration of levodopa to animals (1950s), and Oliver Sacks (the famous neurologist who wrote *The Man Who Mistook His Wife for a Hat*) wrote about the treatment of postencephalitic parkinsonism with levodopa in his book *Awakenings*. Oleh Hornykiewicz, who also played a key role in the development of levodopa, published a recent paper reviewing the discovery of dopamine deficiency (22,26,28,30,33).

What is the best blood test for diagnosing PD?

There is no reliable blood test to diagnose PD. The best way to make a diagnosis is to have a neurological examination by someone experienced in the care of PWPs. There are diagnostic criteria for the diagnosis of PD (UK Brain Bank Criteria), which usually include the following:

I Is bradykinesia (slowness of movement) present?
II Are two of the symptoms given below present?
    (1) Rigidity (stiffness in arms, leg, or neck)
    (2) 4–6 Hertz resting tremor
    (3) Postural instability not caused by primary visual, vestibular, cerebellar, proprioceptive dysfunction
III Are at least three of those mentioned below present?
    (1) Unilateral onset
    (2) Rest tremor
    (3) Progressive disorder
    (4) Persistent asymmetry affecting side of onset most
    (5) Excellent response (70%–100%) to levodopa
    (6) Severe levodopa-induced dyskinesia
    (7) Levodopa response for five years or more
    (8) Clinical course of five years or more

Very rarely, there exists confusion about the diagnosis, and in these cases other tests such as positron emission tomography (PET) scan and beta single photon emission computed tomography (SPECT) scanning may be useful (4,11,37–39).

What sort of training should my doctor have?

The best possible scenario for a PWP is to receive regular care from a neurologist who has completed fellowship training (1–3 years following successful completion of a neurology residency training program) in PD and movement disorders. Currently there is a worldwide shortage of these specialists, and therefore the next best alternative is to seek a general neurologist. When selecting a general neurologist we suggest choosing someone with either a practice focused on PD (or movement disorders), or a neurologist with a special interest in PD. It is important that your doctor takes an interest in you and that he or she is willing to spend more than the average amount of time for a patient visit. We find at minimum, a newly diagnosed PWP may require an hour or more of time and on return visits approximately 30 minutes. Even if your doctor does not possess specialty training, if he or she takes an interest in your case and in this disease, you will likely experience a successful long-term interaction.

We have also found that the best care for a PWP occurs when a complete multi/interdisciplinary team is involved (neurologist, counseling psychologist, neuropsychologist, psychiatrist, speech pathologist, physical therapist, occupational therapist, social worker, etc.). A team working together will have improved communication and will be in a better position to tailor therapies for individual patients.

Can I have a specialty neurologist participate in my care along with a general neurologist/general practitioner?

The best situation for patients is to have both a specialty-trained neurologist (perhaps even at a center of excellence for PD) as well as either a general neurologist or a general medical practitioner. Worldwide, most people may be surprised to learn that general practitioners take care of the majority of PWPs. We advocate for patients to seek outstanding local care (with approximately quarterly visits) and to have specialty care at least once or twice a year. The specialist can help to co-manage the patient and also to inform the patient and the family of new therapies and clinical trials. In addition, when the specialty movement disorders neurologist writes a letter summarizing the findings and management, this can also serve as an educational tool for the general neurologist or practitioner who can apply recommendations and use the added information to improve care paradigms and strategies for shared patients (and future patients).

What is PD really?

PD is a slowly progressive neurodegenerative disorder. Neurodegenerative means that brain cells and brain systems are dying or being lost. The degeneration occurs in multiple brain circuits, and these circuits control both motor and nonmotor functions. In addition, many chemicals in the brain are involved, so it is not just a disease of the chemical dopamine.

In addition to the common motor symptoms (tremor, stiffness, gait problems, slowness, etc.) there can be a multitude of nonmotor manifestations including memory problems, thinking problems, fatigue, mood disturbances (depression, anxiety, mania, and others), sexual dysfunction, constipation, and drooling (as well as a host of other potential symptoms). Many people place a heavy focus on only the motor dysfunction, but in real life the nonmotor symptoms may impact quality of life more than the easily noticeable motor issues like tremor, stiffness, slowness, and shuffling feet (3,11,12,17).

Who gets PD? Is it genetic?

Age is the most prominent risk factor for the development of PD. We like to tell people that if the neuroscientists realize their dream and make everyone live forever, we may all end up with PD.

The simple truth is that anyone can get it, and even though the worldwide average age is in the mid-fifties to early sixties, it can occur at any age. Men are more likely to be affected with PD than women.

PD is probably not one disease. It is likely a syndrome with multiple diseases that share common clinical symptoms (tremor, stiffness, slowness, nonmotor features). There are now several families that have been identified as having a single gene as the responsible factor for their PD. These single gene defects or abnormalities in the DNA (DNA is the word we use to refer to each person's individual genetic makeup) to date account for less than 10% of all cases. The most common and publicized gene defects include LRRK2 and PARKIN (40–46). Gene tests are not in wide commercial use, and those people and families who choose to have a gene test should meet with a genetic counselor. The implications of knowing that you are gene positive for a disease that may strike at any age can result in serious and life-changing implications. In Huntington's disease, where 50% of all children with one parent carrying the disease will become afflicted/affected, only (approximately) half of these patients will ask for a genetic test following genetic counseling. The most widely publicized recent case was that of Segey Brin, the cofounder of Google. After learning that his mom had PD, he and his mom were both tested; Sergey himself was found to be gene positive. Though he does not have any symptoms, there is every likelihood that at some point in future he will develop PD. He has dedicated much of his time and resources to screening for (23 and me), preventing, and treating a disease he will eventually personally suffer from.

The new paradigm in thinking about genetics is that it is more than just an abnormality in DNA. There is likely a complex interaction between the gene and the environment. Some experts have playfully referred to this as the gene loading the gun and the environment pulling the trigger.

There is an outstanding lay review of PD genetics on the website called Genetics Home Reference, produced by the National Library of Medicine. On this site they detail information such as the gene mutations that seem to cause PD—LRRK2, PARK2, PARK7, PINK1, and SNCA—as well as genes associated with PD—GBA, SNCAIP, and UCHL1. The home reference notes that how genes cause disease is unknown, but they offer the following insight:

> ...some mutations appear to disturb the cell machinery that breaks down (degrades) unwanted proteins. As a result, un-degraded proteins accumulate, leading to the impairment or death of dopamine-producing neurons. Other mutations may involve mitochondria, the energy-producing structures within cells. As a by-product of energy production, mitochondria make unstable molecules, called free radicals, that can damage the cell. Normally, the cell neutralizes free radicals, but some gene mutations may disrupt this neutralization process. As a result, free radicals may accumulate and impair or kill dopamine-producing neurons.

So far we believe that LRRK2 and SNCA require the parent to pass only one copy of the gene to the child for inheritance (autosomal dominant). Two copies (one from each parent) seem to be required for PARK2, PARK7, and PINK1 (autosomal recessive). We are still researching inheritance patterns of genetic forms of PD (41,43–44).

What are the risk factors for the development of PD?

There is a branch of medical research called epidemiology. In epidemiological studies, scientists will often go door to door to identify how many people in a population do and do not have a disease. They will then assemble lists of disease characteristics and potential risk factors for a particular disease or syndrome. PD seems to be more common in men than in women but is similar in incidence across many continents, races, and ethnicities. There may be a lower prevalence of PD among African Americans, and this is a point under intensive study.

Risk factors associated with the development of PD (and parkinsonism) include such things as well water, rural living, herbicides/pesticides, trauma, drugs, and exposure to chemicals such as tetrahydroquinolone (found in foods such as barbeque). Head trauma, welding, and several other controversial risk factors have been debated by the experts. The herbicide rotenone has been used to develop animal models of PD as has been the accidentally discovered recreational drug compound referred to as MPTP (1-methyl-4-phenyl-1,2,3,6-tetrahydropyridine). Some studies have pointed to protective factors against the development of PD such as caffeine, nonsteroidal anti-inflammatories, and smoking (1,47–55).

It is important that people suffering from PD understand that risk factors are just risk factors, and once you have been diagnosed with PD, modification of your lifestyle will likely have no impact on these areas. In addition, it is important to realize that there are many epidemiological studies, and sometimes there are conflicts in findings. These conflicts can sometimes be explained by study design, biases (eg, cultural, racial, gender, geographical, etc.), and other factors.

What will be the burden of PD on the planet in 10–20 years?

Dorsey and colleagues recently examined what the burden of PD on the planet will be in 2025. They projected the number of individuals with PD in "Western Europe's 5 most and the world's 10 most populous nations." Dorsey estimated that the "number of individuals with Parkinson's disease over the age of 50 in these countries alone was between 4.1 and 4.6 million in 2005 and it will double to between 8.7 and 9.3 million by 2030." China will have the world's largest burden, but the United States will also grow tremendously (56). In addition, it should be kept in mind that these numbers do not include the many cases that occur before the age of 50.

Is it true that the best experimental animal model of PD was discovered accidentally as a result of recreational drug use?

The drug MPTP was discovered accidentally because a group of recreational drug users presented to a California hospital after taking MPTP instead of the designer drug MPPP. Barry Kidston, a 23-year-old chemistry graduate student injected himself with MPPP and developed symptoms similar to PD. A similar scenario played out in 1982 when, in Santa Clara County, California, seven people suffered a similar fate as Kidston. Dr. William Langston performed a brilliant bit of detective work to track down the cause (The Case of the Frozen Addicts, 1995), and later along with other scientists he developed and perfected the best animal model of PD in existence, the MPTP monkey. Had it not been for this discovery, we would certainly not be as far in PD research (47–48).

What is the link between yawning and dopamine?

The phenomenon of levodopa and dopamine agonists producing a yawn has been well described. Many clever practitioners such as Joe Friedman at Brown University have used this response as a hint as to when their patients are "turning on" (medications kicking in). The response has also interestingly been seen in animals, particularly rats (57–59).

The PWPs yawn as a sign that they are turning on and ready for action. The history of the yawn is quite interesting. Schillar reviewed the topic in a recent paper for the medical literature. Schillar wrote in his abstract on the topic:

> . . . since antiquity yawning has attracted a moderate interest among philosophers, psychologists, physiologists, as well as educators, moralists and physicians. Organisms from birds to men and from the womb to the deathbed were found to be displaying it. While sometimes satisfying to the producer, its display is offensive to the lay observer. Hippocrates had it on his lists of useful 'natures.' Aristotle dropped a few words on the matter. Boerhaave elevated its function to the intellect of animals. Haller has commented on its relation to the acoustic system, blood-flow, and baby sleep. Darwin mentioned it in connection with emotional behavior. Some modern authors praised its beneficial effects on respiration and smell. In the 1960s, Ashley Montagu tried to correct the contemporary failure to explain the behavior by the fact of raised CO_2 and arterial compression. It also interested some neurologists, especially in its association with the encephalitis lethargica in the 1920s, with 'spasmodic yawning,' with epilepsy, not to speak of hysteria. As to boredom or its stimulus, a 40-page dissertation survives from the court of Frederick the Great of the 18th century condemning idleness, a subject that also inspired Blaise Pascal and William James. But in the Hindu world, public yawning was a religious offense (59).

Should I get a PET or SPECT scan to confirm a diagnosis of PD?

Currently in most cases of PD, PET and SPECT scans are unnecessary for confirmation of the diagnosis, especially if you have seen an expert and you are having a satisfactory response to dopaminergic therapy. In cases where the expert is not sure of the diagnosis, and in cases where potentially risky procedures are being considered (eg, deep brain stimulation surgery), it is reasonable to get a PET and/or SPECT scan. It is important to keep in mind that PET and/or SPECT scans should be performed only by experienced centers that have done a large volume of PD scans, because those centers will possess a large database of normative values that can be used to interpret results.

PET scans (like SPECT scans) look at the function of the brain rather than its anatomy. This is an important characteristic because unlike in strokes and tumors, the brain anatomy of a PWP is largely normal. It is the chemical composition (decrease in dopamine and other chemical substances) that turns up as abnormal in cases of PD.

PET scans (or SPECT scans) use a substance that "tags." The dopamine transporter ligand, for example, is a tag that represents surviving dopaminergic brain neurons (cells). Thus, the more of the picture that "lights up," the more surviving neurons. A decrease in uptake may be interpreted by an expert as representing early brain degeneration.

In PD, there is a pattern of early degeneration (cell loss) in the affected area (referred to as the basal ganglia), and this pattern often starts as unilateral (on one side), posterior (back of the structure), and ventral (deep) and later spreads anterior (forward) and dorsal (shallow). The decrease in uptake on the scan should be interpreted only by comparing to normal age-matched control subjects without diseases (and this helps to determine if the scan is abnormal). There are typical scan patterns that may emerge. The more widespread the decrease in uptake on the scan, the more advanced the PD degeneration.

Interpretations can, however, be tricky. The first determination is whether the scan is normal or abnormal. Next, the expert will determine if the scan follows the pattern of PD. Finally a determination will be made as to how severe the degeneration (cell loss) is. There are only a few centers that regularly perform PET scans for PD, and these centers usually have experts in interpretation. Two centers with leading reputations include Long Island Jewish Hospital in New York (North Shore) and Washington University Hospital in St. Louis.

PET scans are FDA approved for the diagnosis of dementia, but not for the diagnosis of PD. However, if you or your relative has cognitive (thinking) impairment, they can in select cases be ordered to be examined for the presence of Alzheimer's changes. Parkinson's often co-occurs with Alzheimer's. The cost can range from $2500 to $5000.

Recently, it has come to light in studies where experts attempted to diagnose PD very early in its course (within the first year of symptoms) for enrollment into a clinical trial that a subset of patients (who were thought to have PD) had negative PET or SPECT scans. These patients did not develop the symptoms of PD. This fact is humbling and lends credence to the importance of following patients over long periods to ensure both accurate diagnosis and appropriate treatment. There are now new imaging techniques emerging for PD that may allow us to better quantitate nonmotor dysfunction, as well as basal ganglia network abnormalities (60–66).

What are the other disorders that may masquerade as PD?

There are several other disorders and syndromes that may masquerade with symptoms similar to PD. These can vary from endocrinologic issues (eg, hypothyroidism) to stroke, to affective disorders (eg, depression), to drug-induced disorders (eg, tardive parkinsonism caused by compazine/ phenergan/metoclopramide), and even to other neurodegenerative phenomena (eg, progressive supernuclear palsy [PSP]) (67–77).

What is parkinsonism or Parkinson Plus?

Parkinsonism simply refers to persons who have symptoms that look like PD, but after careful scrutiny they are found not to have regular idiopathic PD. The symptoms in many cases may include the same motor and non-motor manifestations of PD.

Parkinsonism usually does not respond well to dopamine or to other medications commonly used to treat PD, and your doctor should perform an on/off clinical examination with a tool called the Unified Parkinson's Disease Rating Scale to observe whether there is an adequate response to dopaminergic medications (usually approximately 30% or more in PD).

There are several parkinsonian syndromes, which have distinctive characteristics when compared to regular garden variety PD. Some illustrative examples include the following (not all of the below features need to be present for a diagnosis):

- **Lewy body disease:** Parkinson's symptoms plus hallucinations (seeing things that are not present) and thinking problems, which occur within the first few years of diagnosis.
- **Corticobasal degeneration (CBD):** Parkinson's symptoms along with problems with skilled movements (apraxia), a misbehaving limb (alien limb), sensory loss, myoclonus (sudden lightening-like movements), and possibly dementia.
- **Mutiple system atrophy (MSA)—cerebellar type:** Parkinson's symptoms plus problems walking and problems with coordination (also called olivopontocerebellar degeneration [OPCA]).
- **MSA—autonomic type:** Parkinson's symptoms plus problems with autonomic dysfunction (early erectile or sexual dysfunction, dizziness when standing up, problems with digestion and/or constipation [also referred to sometimes as Shy-Drager syndrome]).
- **MSA—striatonigral degeneration type:** Severe Parkinson's symptoms but largely unresponsive to dopaminergic therapy.
- **PSP:** Severe Parkinson's symptoms, plus early falling, dementia, and problems moving the eyes particularly in the up and down directions.
- **Vascular parkinsonism:** Usually presents with shuffling feet (some people call it lower-body parkinsonism) and it is usually caused by small strokes with or without other Parkinson's symptoms.

We like to conservatively observe regular cases of PD for five or more years before making a definitive diagnosis because in some cases parkinsonism or Parkinson's Plus can be levodopa responsive for many years into the illness (67–77).

What is Lewy body disease and how do you treat it?

Lewy body disease is so named because in the brains of patients with this syndrome, we find deposits of a protein called the Lewy body. A Lewy body is actually present normally in PD brains; but when present throughout multiple brain regions and when patients have cognitive symptoms or early hallucinations within the first several years of treatment we suspect this syndrome. The syndrome often presents with daytime jerking (myoclonus).

Some of the symptoms of Lewy body disease include the following (not all must be present for a diagnosis):

(1) Parkinsonism—stiffness (rigidity), slowness (bradykinesia), tremor, shuffling gait.

(2) The symptoms may be asymmetric meaning one side of the body may be more affected.

(3) There may be no response to dopaminergic medications, worsening with medications, or a negative (paradoxical worsening) response(s) to medications. Many patients with this disorder experience paradoxical (unexpected) worsening with dopamine compounds (and other medications), and many others may actually experience some improvement with dopaminergics.

(4) Early and significant hallucinations, which may or may not be associated with dopamine drugs.

(5) Early cognitive and thinking problems (within the first few years of following the symptoms onset).

(6) Fluctuating levels of attention (may appear normal or more normal at some points in the day, and totally demented or lethargic at other points in the same day).

The pathology (what is seen on brain slices after death) for Lewy body disease can appear similar to PD, and some Lewy body patients in addition also have Alzheimer's disease (AD) pathology.

The Lewy body may be the brain's attempt to throw away bad proteins. These bad proteins accumulate and may end up as deposits in the brain. When we stain these brains (at autopsy) we may find a protein called alpha-synuclein (common in PD) and/or Tau (common in AD).

The treatment for Lewy body disease may include drugs such as Aricept or Exelon (acetycholinesterase types of drugs, which make this important chemical for memory more available), drugs like quetiapine and clozapine for hallucinations/behavioral issues, and careful use of dopaminergics (Sinemet and agonists). Many cases will also require antidepressant therapy for mood disturbances. These patients may also benefit from treatment by a multi/interdisciplinary team (physical therapy, occupational therapy, speech therapy, psychology, etc.) (78–81).

What is MSA (Shy-Drager, OPCA, striatonigral degeneration) and how is it treated?

MSA is a disorder in which symptoms look very similar to PD; however, patients may present with additional disabling features. The disorder seems to be more resistant to treatment with common dopaminergic compounds.

There are three major types of MSA (explained in the earlier description of parkinsonism). All three types share a common pathology (seen in samples taken at autopsy) in the brain. The common deposits are referred to as glial cytoplasmic inclusions (at this time we are not sure why these occur, but they seem to be similar to the inclusions seen in PD—the Lewy bodies). The brains of MSA patients stain for alpha-synuclein, a protein commonly encountered in PD.

MSA patients may initially present with symptoms that are responsive to Sinemet (carbidopa/levodopa), dopamine agonists, and other parkinsonian treatments including therapy administered by a multidisciplinary team (physical therapy, occupational therapy, speech therapy, psychology, etc.). Therefore, MSA patients should be treated similarly to PWPs, unless they cannot tolerate the medications or they derive no clinical benefit from them. Often orthostasis (dizziness when standing up resulting from low blood pressure) presents the most immediate and important problem. Treatment with stockings on the legs, fluids, and in some severe cases with medications may be indicated (to raise the blood pressure—midodrine, florinef, and/or physostigmine). Patients may present with numbness (from neuropathy), and this should be evaluated carefully to search reversible causes (the evaluation is usually performed by a neurologist who may use blood tests and nerve conduction studies). Some patients with MSA present with slurry voices and others present with peculiar breathing patterns. Sexual, gastrointestinal, gait, and other symptoms of MSA should be treated by a multi/interdisciplinary team. Cognitive dysfunction or depression can occur, and consideration of cholinesterase inhibitors and antidepressants should be given especially in the early year(s) treatment strategy (82–84).

What is CBD and how is it treated?

CBD is a form of parkinsonism that looks a lot like PD but is less responsive to treatment and patients may experience a faster disease progression.

Symptoms common to CBD may include the following (not all must be present for diagnosis):

(1) Parkinsonism—stiffness (rigidity), slowness (bradykinesia), tremor, shuffling gait
(2) The symptoms may be asymmetric, meaning that one side of the body may be more affected (especially early in the course).
(3) A misbehaving limb (often called an alien limb) that may grope or perform acts the person may not desire (eg, an arm or leg may levitate uncontrollably, or one arm may pull the pants up, while the other pushes them down).
(4) Loss of sensation or certain types of sensation on one side of the body (cortical sensory loss—cannot identify objects placed in the hand when eyes are closed)
(5) Loss of the ability to perform skilled movements (apraxia)
(6) Possible dementia
(7) Abnormal postures of limbs called dystonia, or abnormal, fast, lightning-like movements referred to as myoclonus.

Some patients with CBD present with parkinsonism, and others present with more prominent dementia without the presence of much parkinsonism.

The pathology (from autopsy samples taken after death) encountered in the brain in CBD is similar to what is found in AD. CBD brains stain with a protein called Tau (as in AD), but have a special finding in the tissue (cells that look like balloons).

The treatment for CBD is the same as that employed for PD, except that the medications often do not work as well, and sometimes can worsen the clinical course. Dopamine, dopamine agonists, antidepressants, cholinesterase inhibitors, and interdisciplinary care (physical therapy, occupational therapy, speech therapy, psychology, psychiatry, etc.) can all be useful (85).

What is Progressive Supranuclear Palsy (PSP) and how is it treated?

PSP is a parkinsonian disorder that has a lot of features that look like PD, but these features usually do not respond well to Sinemet (dopamine) and to other medication therapies.

Common symptoms may include the following:

(1) Parkinsonism—stiffness (rigidity), slowness (bradykinesia), tremor, shuffling gait
(2) Sometimes the symptoms are not as asymmetric as in PD
(3) Early falling (within the first one or two years of onset)
(4) Trouble walking down stairs
(5) Trouble moving the eyes (have to turn the head to look in certain directions, and trouble moving the eyes up and down)
(6) Abnormal postures (dystonia)
(7) A face that looks locked in time, stone face
(8) Cognitive or thinking problems
(9) Emotional ability (pseudobulbar affect or emotional incontinence)—easy crying or laughing

The pathology of PSP (from autopsy samples taken after death) is similar to that encountered in CBD and in AD (the Tau protein deposits in the brain). There is a form of PSP that can be caused by multiple small strokes (vascular PSP), and this can be identified by use of an MRI scan.

We often attempt to treat PSP the same as we treat PD; but most of the symptoms are less responsive and the disease course is faster and in most cases more devastating. Severe drooling and dystonia can be addressed by botulinum toxin therapy (68,76).

What is vascular parkinsonism (lower-body parkinsonism, Binswanger disease, multi-infarct dementia)?

Sometimes parkinsonian symptoms may look like PD and may not respond in a positive way to medications. MRI or CT brain imaging scans may reveal a large number of small strokes (areas where the brain did not get enough oxygen and the cells died) or alternatively a lot of white matter changes. White matter in the brain is a conglomeration of fibers that function to provide the connection between the brain's many islands. The pattern of multiple strokes or of diffuse white matter changes has been referred to as vascular parkinsonism, Binswanger disease, or multi-infarct dementia. It is often, but not always, symmetrical (symptoms are the same on both sides), and it may affect the legs much more than the arms—leading some to call it lower-body parkinsonism. In our experience, it can have a variable spectrum of symptoms beyond solely leg involvement.

The treatment for vascular parkinsonism can be challenging, with preventative therapies for stroke (manage diabetes, high blood pressure, smoking, diet, etc.) providing the best long-term solutions. It is important in these cases to prescribe multi/interdisciplinary services such as physical therapy, occupational therapy, speech therapy, psychology, or psychiatry as needed on an individualized basis depending on the symptom complex.

It is important to keep in mind that many patients will acquire small strokes as they age, and many also have evidence for asymptomatic white matter changes on MRI scan(s) (an MRI or computed tomography [CT] scan is obtained for an unrelated problem such as headache and white matter changes are discovered). It is essential to treat vascular parkinsonian patients with the standard therapies available to regular PWPs, because in many cases they may have both vascular changes and also PD (offer a trial of levodopa) (74).

What is essential tremor and how is it different from PD?

Essential tremor usually occurs when the hands are held at posture (like Superman holds his arms in front of his body) and at action (eg, finger-to-nose maneuvers, during drinking/handwriting). In contrast, PD tremor is more commonly observed at rest (but may be mildly present with posture and action). Both diseases are now considered by many experts to be neurodegenerative disorders (disorders where brain cells die). Essential tremor is more common than PD, and it may affect all ages including young children. In some patients, the tremor improves with alcohol, and practitioners should be cautious in looking for signs and symptoms of alcohol abuse.

The cause of essential tremor is unknown, although it is believed that there exists an abnormal communication in a brain circuit referred to as the cerebello-thalamo-cortical loop. There is currently no known pathology (tissue) finding in essential tremor; however, there is a brain bank that has been formed to search for the possibility of tissue changes. Patients can (late in the course of the disease) experience mild cognitive or thinking problems that may include memory difficulties and what is sometimes referred to as errors or problems in frontal lobe function (sequencing, executive function, initiating behavior, inhibiting behavior). Severe cases may experience difficulty when walking heel to toe (referred to as tandem gait problems). In these cases, the dysfunction is thought to be related to problems in a coordination center in a part of the brain referred to as the cerebellum. Patients may also experience voice, tongue, and/or lip tremors.

The main disability in essential tremor is derived from the action tremor, which can in severe cases make handwriting, eating, and performing activities of daily living nearly impossible.

Treatments include an anticonvulsant called primidone (mysoline), beta-blockers (eg, propranolol and other medications ending in the letters "ol"), and benzodiazepines (clonazepam, valium, etc.). If the tremor is disabling and fails to respond to medications, then thalamic deep brain stimulation (DBS) or lesion therapy in select cases may be a very effective treatment (86–89).

Are there other brain lesions that can cause tremor and be confused with PD?

A tremendous number of reports of brain lesions resulting in tremor have been described in the literature, so one should not automatically assume PD or essential tremor when shaking is encountered. Recent advances in imaging capabilities and advances in other diagnostic techniques have propelled the recognition and reporting of a myriad of diseases and pathologies that may affect multiple brain regions. These abnormalities can result in almost every type of tremor disorder. State-of-the-art MRI scans may expose a lesion's anatomical devastation, which may translate into abnormal communication between brain islands and consequently tremor. Pressure effects of brain lesions on the contiguous or contralateral (other side of the brain) areas may also explain a patient's tremor. Only recent case reports have considered the vascular effects of intracranial lesions on distant brain regions, and many of these reports have utilized a new relatively new technology called magnetic resonance angiography (MRA). Tremor can also result from intracranial, infectious, and neoplastic (cancer) lesions, slow infiltration, coinfection, edema (swelling), distant metastasis (spread of cancer), and antibody/paraneoplastic phenomena (the body's immune response to a cancer).

In addition, a variety of treatments have been utilized to control tremors resulting from cerebral lesions. These treatments have widely variable success rates. Descriptions of tremor treatment success and failure largely depend on the prognosis and treatment of the primary etiology as well as the degree of functional disability encountered from the tremor. In some cases, tremor is only an incidental finding in a more malignant syndrome, while in other cases it is the presenting or most disabling feature. Every pharmacological option is usually sought as first-line therapy, especially if surgical resection of a primary brain lesion (if present) is not possible.

Different tremors may respond to individualized and very specific treatments. Drugs such as carbidopa/levodopa, dopamine agonists, anticholinergics, amantadine, clozapine, anticonvulsants, and other pharmacologic agents may be attempted. There are reports that reveal variable successes with these drugs when individualized for specific tremor disorders. DBS and surgical lesion therapy may be an option in some tremor subtypes that prove resistant to medicines (89,90–94).

What is AD, and can it cooccur with PD?

AD, like PD, is a neurodegenerative disorder (cells dying in the brain) that can lead to memory loss, confusion, hallucinations, behavioral disorders, and difficulty in thinking. A large percentage of patients with AD can have features that appear similar to PD (stiffness, slowness, tremor, or gait problems), which is why it is important to visit a movement disorders neurologist or a neurologist with some expertise in PD or neurodegenerative disorders—to obtain the correct diagnosis and consequently appropriate treatment. PD can co-occur with AD (some call it PD/AD), and this can present unique treatment challenges (eg, medication sensitivity, increased memory and cognitive problems, or difficult-to-control hallucinations).

AD seems to be associated with deposition in the brain of the Tau protein, while PD is associated with deposition of alpha-synuclein.

Current symptomatic treatments for AD may include the use of a multi/interdisciplinary team, cholinesterase inhibitors (these stimulate a chemical called acetylcholine, which may improve memory), Memantine (stimulates a chemical called glutamate, which is important for learning and thinking), as well as the provision of behavioral training and education for affected families. The same therapies may also be applied to PWPs with cognitive problems (95,96).

How should I treat difficult-to-control tremor associated with PD?

Tremor that does not respond completely, or satisfactorily (improves the symptoms, so quality of life's activities are no longer impaired), to the standard PD medications may occur in a significant proportion of sufferers (approximately 20%–40%). One approach to this problem has been to offer a cocktail of medications that may in synergy be more effective than any single agent. We recommend that practitioners should start with one medication, increase the dose to a maximally tolerated level, then add a second, a third, and potentially even a fourth medication if necessary. One common strategy is to start with Sinemet (carbidopa/levodopa) 25/100 and take the pills every 3, 4, or 5 hours (on a religious time interval). The dose should be increased gradually as tolerated to a maximum of 2.5 to 3 pills at each interval. Then, one may add a dopamine agonist, usually pramipexole (3–5 mg/day divided doses) or ropinirole (20–24 mg/day in divided doses). The maximally tolerated doses of both Sinemet and the dopamine agonist should be maintained together in case the cocktail offers synergy (more benefit with the combination compared to either one of the drugs alone). If tremor remains a problem, trihexyphenidyl, benztropine, or ethopropazine can be added. These three medications are in a class called anticholinergics and should be used cautiously as side effects such as drowsiness, confusion, memory loss, blurry vision, or bladder difficulties may be associated with their use. After attempting this cocktail of three drugs, if tremor is still bothersome, some practitioners add a beta-blocker, anticonvulsant, or amantadine. The last resort of medication for refractory tremor with or without motor fluctuations would be DBS or lesion therapy (for well-selected and well-screened patients) (86,89,92,93).

I was just diagnosed with PD and I get nausea every time I try to start my PD medications, what should I do?

Dopamine and dopaminergics when taken orally (by mouth) may commonly result in nausea especially when the body is first exposed to them. Nausea therefore should not be an automatic reason for discontinuation of dopaminergic drugs.

In the case of Sinemet (carbidopa/levodopa), the drug must cross the blood-brain barrier to stimulate the dopaminergic brain system and to achieve the intended effects of dopamine replacement. Dopamine circulates in the peripheral blood and may stimulate a brain center that is not protected by the blood-brain barrier (the area postrema). This brain center when stimulated will result in the subjective sensation of nausea and sometimes even lead to vomiting. Straight dopamine will not effectively cross the blood-brain barrier. We therefore pair dopamine with a drug called carbidopa or a drug used in Europe called benzerazide. These drugs are designed to block an enzyme called dopamine decarboxylase that breaks down dopamine. We give L-dopa instead of dopamine, as L-dopa will cross the blood-brain barrier. By preventing conversion peripherally to dopamine, carbidopa, and benzerazide prevent the stimulation of nausea centers in the brain.

Patients with Sinemet-induced nausea can be prescribed extra doses of carbidopa in an attempt to block more dopamine decarboxylase and consequently reduce nausea. The brain may over the course of weeks to months develop tolerance to Sinemet, and the extra carbidopa may prove unnecessary.

Dopamine agonist–induced nausea is much more difficult to treat because dopamine agonists go directly to brain dopamine receptors and stimulate them, which leaves the practitioner with fewer options for treatment. The best treatment in dopamine agonist–induced nausea therefore may be a very slow titration onto the drug allowing the brain time to adjust and develop tolerance. In many cases, patients may simply not tolerate dopamine agonists because of nausea.

Finally, nausea may also be treated by a drug called domperidone (not the champagne). Domperidone is a very powerful dopamine blocker that does not cross the blood-brain barrier. We try never to use dopamine blockers that cross the blood-brain barrier in PD as they may worsen symptoms. Common drugs used for headache and gastrointestinal disease such as compazine, phenergan, and metoclopramide block dopamine and worsen PD and therefore are relatively contraindicated. Therefore, if another nausea drug is required, we strongly advocate domperidone, or alternatively ondansetron (Zofran), which works on a different brain system and will suppress nauseous feelings (97–100).

I experience inappropriate crying and laughing spells; can that be PD?

We recently examined this question of inappropriate laughing and crying in PD and other movement disorders. In the study, we examined inappropriate crying and laughing and underlying mood disturbances in a large clinic-based population of PD and movement disorder patients. PBA is characterized by uncontrollable laughter without mirth, or alternatively crying without the feeling of sadness. It is a common condition affecting more than one million people with neurological diseases. While PBA has been studied in many neurological diseases, little is known about its prevalence in movement disorders or its relationship to more chronic mood disturbances. In all, 719 out of 860 consecutive patients who visited our Movement Disorders Center met criteria for the study and were interviewed for symptoms of PBA during their visit. In addition, 661 of these patients completed both the visual analog mood scale (VAMS) and beck depression inventory-I (BDI-I). In all, 37 of the 719 reported PBA symptoms: 75.7% (28/37) had pathological crying, 13.5% (5/37) had pathological laughing, and 10.8% (4/37) had both. The prevalence of PBA in individual diagnostic categories was: (a) 4.7% (18/387) of idiopathic PD, (b) 2.7% (2/74) of primary dystonia, (c) 3.1% (2/65) of essential tremor (ET), (d) 7.8% (8/108) of patients with other forms of parkinsonism, (e) 21.7% (5/23) of psychogenic movement disorders, (f) 0% (0/18) of patients with combined PD and ET, and (g) 4.5% (2/44) of other movement disorders. Patients with PBA had a higher total BDI depression score and VAMS "tiredness" score. PBA was present in most movement disorders but prevalent especially in parkinsonism. PBA patients in this cohort had more chronic depressive symptoms and tiredness. In addition, we have reported PBA following Parkinson lesion surgery (thalamotomy) and following DBS. In most cases, it is easily treatable with a low dose of an antidepressant (101–103).

Is vision impaired in PD?

Visual activity is usually not impaired tremendously in PD, although some-times seeing contrast in color, color vision, and visuospatial processing may be affected. What is most commonly impaired is the ability of the eyes to work together. What may happen is that the person with PD develops what is called convergence insufficiency, and this leads to double vision particularly when things are held closer to the eyes. Solutions to vision problems in PD may include prisms and holding books and objects further from the eyes. Vision issues can also include problems with depth percep-tion that can affect reaction time and driving ability as well (104,105).

Biousse and colleagues studied ophthalmological issues in PWPs. These authors discovered that when compared to patients without PD, the disease cohort had more ocular complaints including ocular surface irri-tation, altered tear film, visual hallucinations, blepharospasm, decreased blink rate, and decreased convergence amplitudes. They hypothesized that these issues may contribute to the visual complaints in PWPs (106). There are many other potential causes of visual problems not related to PD, and we therefore always recommend a neuro-opthalmological examination for any eye-related difficulties.

Is there a cure for PD?

Despite many television, Internet, and print offers that tout a fee-for-cure therapeutic regimen for PD, there is currently no known cure for this condition.

I don't have a tremor, can I still have PD?

Studies have been performed that have revealed there are many subtypes of PD. These subtypes may include tremor-dominant, akinetic-rigid, and postural-instability gait subtype(s). It is estimated that one in five PWPs do not suffer from tremor. Therefore, the absence of tremor does not exclude the possibility of PD (37–39,107–110).

What parts of the brain degenerate (die) in PD?

There has been a long-held belief among physicians and scientists that the only part of the brain to die in PD are the small pigmented brain cells in the brainstem called the substantia nigra, or black substance. We now know that this view was myopic and too simplistic. There are multiple circuits in the brain that degenerate in PD. These circuits are referred to as the basal ganglia, and they include such structures as the globus palli-dus, subthalamic nucleus, thalamus, and cerebral cortex. There are motor, nonmotor, and eye circuits that degenerate. Depending on the areas of degeneration, PWPs may experience different disease manifestations relative to the brain dysfunction.

On a typical brain CT or MRI, it is difficult to see the pathology underlying PD. However, by cutting donated postmortem (after death) brains of PWPs we have been able to visualize the dysfunction by the use of tissue stains and microscopes. There is an abnormal protein called alpha-synuclein that can be stained and visualized by light microscopy. Similarly, we find a protein that is deposited into brain tissues that is referred to as a Lewy body (named after Professor Lewy). Braak and colleagues studied hundreds of PD brains and they recently proposed a staging system. In their scheme, PD is proposed to actually start two stages before involvement of the substantia nigra cells in the midbrain. They propose the dysfunction may start in autonomic and lower brainstem systems and progress upward or rostral toward the cerebral cortex. The idea is that as the PD spreads rostrally, so too do the clinical symptoms. This is a provocative theory, which has yet to be completely accepted (16,17,20,21,111,112).

What are the main theories for the cause of PD?

There are many theories as to the cause of PD. These include (a) synucleinopathy (deposition of proteins), (b) excitotoxicity (too much of a chemical called glutamate which may be excitotoxic), (c) calcium homeostasis (calcium-related enzymes may get activated and lead to brain cell death), (d) mitochondrial-related cell death (the mitochondria are the power plants for each cell in the brain and may be abnormal in PD), and (e) inflammation. Each of these proposed theories has led to the independent search for therapeutic treatment targets.

It has also been proposed that oxidative stress, mitochondrial dysfunction, excitotoxicity, and inflammation together contribute to problems with protein handling in the brain and also contribute to the formation of Lewy bodies. These processes may lead to further brain neuronal dysfunction and death of cells.

It is widely viewed by many experts that degenerative disorders such as PD result from a cascade of abnormalities that ultimately result in abnormal protein processing and consequent disease symptoms. At this time, all these suppositions remain speculative with varying degrees of scientific evidence to support their basis (113–123).

What is normal pressure hydrocephalus and should I worry about it?

Normal pressure hydrocephalus (NPH) is a brain condition that occurs when there is an excessive accumulation of cerebrospinal fluid (this is the fluid that the brain and spinal cord normally bathe in by utilizing a system in the brain called the ventricles). When the reservoirs (also known as the ventricles) that carry the brain fluid enlarge, they can stretch brain structures and put them under pressure. This pressure can result in symptoms such as cognitive dysfunction, walking problems, and incontinence (sometimes referred to as the triad of whacky, wobbly, and wet). As the name infers that although enlarged, the actual pressure measured in the ventricular system is completely normal. Unfortunately, recent studies have refuted that the pressure is normal in NPH, making the name a misnomer.

There has unfortunately been a lot of confusion between NPH and PD. One of the reasons for the confusion is that in PD the ventricles are often big and therefore may be mistaken for NPH. Therefore, one clinical pearl is to always try levodopa, which may be one of several ways to help differentiate the two (67,124–126).

Should a plan be in place if I am hospitalized with PD?

Most people with PD will need to be hospitalized at some time. Common reasons for hospital admissions from the emergency room can include infections of the urinary tract or lung (such as pneumonia), chest pain, heart failure, falls, and psychiatric issues. Common reasons for non-emergent hospitalizations include elective surgeries such as knee and hip replacements. Hospitalization can be stressful for a number of important reasons. The neurologist who takes care of you and manages your PD medications may not have privileges at the hospital where you are admitted, and the physicians responsible for your care in the hospital may not know a lot about PD. Furthermore, the nursing staff may not have much experience with patients who have your symptoms and will likely have little time to invest in learning for various reasons including nursing shortages and/or cuts in staffing. Finally, if you need to undergo surgery or other invasive medical procedures, you may not be able to take any medications until the surgery or procedure is complete. It is important for the patient and the caregiver to plan and to anticipate what is likely to happen. The combination of education and planning can alleviate many of the problems encountered in the hospital (127).

When I am in the hospital, why don't I always get my medications on time?

It is important to realize that hospitals and hospital pharmacies have their own dosing schedules. For example, if a medication is written for "QID (four times a day)," the standard hospital schedule may be 8 AM–1 PM– 6 PM–11 PM or some similar variation. A medication written for "TID (three times a day)" may be given at 7 AM–3 PM–11 PM or some other standard schedule. Furthermore, many hospitals may have a policy where the nurses have a window where they can give medications (generally, one hour before the scheduled time to one hour after the scheduled time). This window is provided as a practical compromise because nursing staffs are busy, and each nurse usually cares for multiple patients. Such a policy provides the nurse time to complete his/her scheduled duties and provides flexibility in case of emergency on the ward. As a result, PWPs will in most cases receive their medications at seemingly random times.

How can such a situation be remedied? First, make sure that the drug schedule, with specific times, is written into the doctor's orders. For example, if carbidopa/levodopa (Sinemet) is given four times a day, but at 6 AM–10 AM–2 PM–6 PM, make sure that the physician taking care of you knows that it should be given at those specific times. Also, make sure that you bring with you the complete list of your medications and the dose of each medication is correct. Carbidopa/levodopa can come as a 10/100, 25/100, or 25/250 tablet for the standard form, while the long-acting form (Sinemet CR) comes in two strengths, 25/100 and 50/200. Other common medications, such as pramipexole (Mirapex) and ropinirole (Requip), also come in multiple strengths. Finally, when you first arrive in your room, talk with your nurse about the importance of receiving your medications on time. Explain that without the medications you can be immobile or uncomfortable and that the medications allow you to move around independently. You may know more about PD than the doctor and the staff, and it is your job to help them understand your situation. While you will still need to be somewhat flexible (there are many other important things that may occupy a nurse's time), sharing your knowledge with the staff can alleviate many problems. All hospital staffs want their patients to be well cared for during their stay.

Not everyone in the hospital has experience treating PWPs, so you should share your knowledge and help them understand why you need to take your medications at specific times (127).

Why can't I take my own medications in the hospital? Why do they substitute some medications for me?

While you are hospitalized, the nursing staff must have control of your medications. This is a safety issue and is standard hospital policy. It is not a reflection of what the staff thinks of you, so do not take it personally. If you let the staff know what is supposed to be given and how it is to be administered, there should not be any significant problems.

In some cases, patients may be taking medications that are not stocked in the hospital pharmacy. In such situations, the physician taking care of you in the hospital may have to prescribe substitute medications. If you want to take your own medications, you need to bring them from home in their original bottles and give them to the nursing staff. They will then dispense your medications while you are admitted, and there will be no need for substitution. If you are enrolled in an experimental drug protocol, it is even more important that you follow this practice. In some hospitals and outpatient surgical facilities, the doctor can write an order to allow patients to take their own medicines; however, the doses and times must be written in the chart and the pill ingestion must be supervised and documented.

Find out the hospital rule on taking your own medication. Always bring your medications in the original bottles along with a list of the medications, doses, and times of administration (127).

My mother has PD and was recently hospitalized. However, she seems to be moving much worse in the hospital than at home. Why is that?

Several explanations are possible. When patients with PD have an infection of some kind, whether it is the common cold, pneumonia, or a urinary tract infection, they often feel like their symptoms worsen. Increased tremor or more difficulty walking may be noted. When the infection is treated and resolves, the symptoms generally return to baseline. Another symptom that may worsen when PWPs have an infection is swallowing. When swallowing is impaired and patients are weak, the food may go down into the lungs, causing an aspiration pneumonia, which in turn, may further impair swallowing ability. In these situations, a speech pathology consultation can be useful to formally assess swallowing and make dietary recommendations. In addition, a respiratory therapist consultation for chest physical therapy (PT) may be helpful. Chest PT consists of several minutes of chest clapping to help mobilize the sputum and make it easier to cough.

Another possibility is new medication. Common offenders include antipsychotic drugs or antinausea drugs. Haloperidol (Haldol) is a common antipsychotic drug that is used in hospital settings. This drug blocks dopamine receptors and worsens PD. Other commonly used antipsychotics include risperidone (Risperdal), olanzapine (Zyprexa), and aripiprazole (Abilify). The only antipsychotics that can be used safely in PWPs are clozapine (Clozaril) and quetiapine (Seroquel). Common antinausea medications that can worsen symptoms of PD include prochlorperazine

(Compazine), promethazine (Phenergan), and metoclopramide (Reglan). These medications have similar structures to the antipsychotics and should not be used. Trimethobenzamide (Tigan) and ondansetron (Zofran) are suitable alternatives that can be used without fear of worsening symptoms.

Regardless of the cause, all PWPs should be as active as possible while in the hospital. Moving around not only tones muscle, it allows faster recovery and prevents decomposition of the skin, which can happen when staying in one position for too long. Depending upon your condition, however, you may not have a choice, and your doctor may order you to bed rest. In that case, physical therapy should be ordered as soon as possible. Some patients may also need rehabilitation at a rehabilitation hospital or a nursing facility before being discharged to home.

There are multiple explanations for worsening of PD while in the hospital. Infections should be sought and treated. Drugs that block dopamine, like haloperidol and certain antinausea drugs, should be avoided. Chest PT, speech pathology, and physical therapy may all be useful in the recovery process (127).

My husband has PD and became confused in the hospital last time he was there. How can I prevent this?

Many things happen in the hospital that can contribute to confusion. Any infection in a PWP can be enough to tip a patient over the edge mentally. Similarly, infections can adversely affect motor function as we discussed earlier. The introduction of new medications frequently results in disorientation and memory problems, especially pain medications. Lack of sleep while in the hospital can also contribute to a confusional state. Continuous alarms from intravenous machines and hallway lights can all result in frequent awakening. Nurses also may regularly enter the room overnight to take vital signs, give medications, or to check on a patient. In some patients, especially in the elderly with intermittent confusion at home, just the fact that they are placed in a different and unfamiliar environment may tip them into a delirious state. Finally, confusion is commonly seen following a surgical procedure. The combined effects of anesthesia and medications to treat surgical incision pain are contributing factors in this situation.

Confusion will often disappear once the underlying cause is treated, whether it is addressing the infection or withdrawing the offending medications. Diagnostic testing is rarely necessary. Frequent reassurance, support, and comfort may be all that is needed to assist the patient through this period. However, sometimes confusion can lead to behavioral problems, such as aggression, refusal to take pills, and even hallucinations or delusions. In these cases, physical restraints are sometimes necessary to prevent self-injury. Some hospitals have bed or wheelchair alarms to alert nurses when patients attempt to wander, while other hospitals may use a sitter to promote safety. If there are psychotic symptoms, such as visual hallucinations, antipsychotics may be used. Remember in nearly all cases, clozapine (Clozaril) and quetiapine (Seroquel) are the only antipsychotics that should be used in PWPs. Occasionally, lorazepam (Ativan) or diazepam (Valium) can be helpful. These drugs, by themselves, may worsen confusion, but they also can calm the patient. These medications are only temporary and may be discontinued when the confusion resolves.

In very severe cases of confusion with hallucinations and behavioral changes, it may be necessary to temporarily discontinue dopamine agonists, manoamine oxidase (MAO) inhibitors, amantadine, benzodiazepines, and pain medications if possible. Treatment with carbidopa/levodopa and either clozapine or quetiapine will usually result in improvement. Later, once patients are stable, they may be slowly titrated back onto previous doses if tolerated (127).

Infection and medications are common causes of confusion in the hospital, and when the underlying cause is addressed, it usually improves dramatically.

I had DBS placed two years ago. I now need to have knee replacement surgery. Will the doctors know how to take care of me?

While thousands of patients worldwide have had DBS treatment for PD and other movement disorders, many medical professionals and hospitals may still not be familiar with this treatment. Many patients with DBS undergo knee replacement surgery and other procedures without difficulty. However, there are a few things you and your doctors should be aware of. First of all, if you have had DBS surgery, you can only get an MRI of the brain, and it must be done with something called a head-receive coil. You cannot get an MRI of any other part of the body. This situation exists because the DBS device can become heated and damage the brain tissue during MRI. There are also certain precautions that the radiologists must be aware of while performing a brain MRI. These are available from the FDA. Furthermore, the voltage on your stimulator should be turned down to zero prior to having an MRI performed. Only an experienced programmer should supervise the procedure. If an experienced member of the DBS team is not available in the hospital where you are being treated, and/or if the institution is not familiar with performing

MRIs in DBS patients, it is probably best not to have the MRI, or to wait and have it at an experienced center.

The stimulators can sometimes interfere with the ability to obtain an electrocardiogram (ECG). This test may be important if you happen to have cardiac problems before, during, or after surgery. Therefore, you should bring your portable Medtronic access device or access review device (or a magnet that comes with the device) to turn off your stimulator in the hospital. Make sure you know how to turn your stimulators on and off before going to the hospital and before having any type of surgery. (Again, do not assume that the medical staff will be able to turn them off for you.) Similarly, if you need a brain wave test called an electroencephalogram (EEG), or if you will simply be monitored during an inpatient or outpatient procedure you will need to know how to turn your device off.

If you are undergoing surgery and you have DBS, most anesthetics are safe. However, some precautions need to be taken when using electrocautery. Electrocautery stops bleeding during surgery and could potentially reset your stimulator to its factory settings. As a precaution, only bipolar electrocautery is recommended (with grounding placed below the level of the device). If your neurologist is on staff at the hospital where you are getting surgery, he or she should confirm that your stimulator is on and that the correct settings are reset following surgery. If your neurologist is not at the hospital where you are having surgery, you should schedule a follow-up appointment soon after you are discharged from the hospital to recheck your settings.

Be aware of what procedures can be done safely with DBS, and be ready to assume primary responsibility for turning it on and off for procedures.

Be aware that for unclear reasons some symptoms worsen following general or local anesthesia, some patients have even reported feeling as if they never return to their baseline. In general, local anesthesia is thought to be safer than general anesthesia, and if you have problems with thinking and memory, they should be evaluated prior to surgery as they may also worsen (127).

How can I be sure my wishes will be honored in case something unexpected and bad happens during my hospitalization?

It is important for you to have discussions with close family members about what you would like to have done in case of a life-threatening emergency. They and the medical staff should be aware of your medical wishes. You should choose an advocate who can ask questions and act as your spokesperson. If you have a living will or a durable health care power of attorney, these documents should be brought to the hospital and placed in the medical chart.

FURTHER READING

DATATOP: a multicenter controlled clinical trial in early Parkinson's disease. Parkinson Study Group. *Arch Neurol.* 1989;46(10):1052–1060.

Castro A, Valldeoriola F, Linazasoro G, et al. (2005). Optimization of use of levodopa in Parkinson's disease: role of levodopa-carbidopa-entacapone combination [in Spanish]. *Neurologia.* 20(4):180–188.

Chan PL, Nutt JG, Holford NH. Levodopa slows progression of Parkinson's disease: external validation by clinical trial simulation. *Pharm Res.* 2007;24(4):791–802.

Clarke CE. Neuroprotection and pharmacotherapy for motor symptoms in Parkinson's disease. *Lancet Neurol.* 2004;3(8):466–474.

Fahn S. Does levodopa slow or hasten the rate of progression of Parkinson's disease? *J Neurol.* 2005;252(suppl 4):IV37–IV42.

Fahn S. A new look at levodopa based on the ELLDOPA study. *J Neural Transm Suppl.* 2006;(70):419–426.

Fahn S. Levodopa in the treatment of Parkinson's disease. *J Neural Transm Suppl.* 2006;(71):1–15.

Fernandez HH, Chen JJ. Monamine oxidase inhibitors: current and emerging agents for Parkinson disease. *Clin Neuropharmacol.* 2007;30(3):150–168.

Fernandez HH, Chen JJ. Monoamine oxidase-B inhibition in the treatment of Parkinson's disease. *Pharmacotherapy.* 2007;27(12, pt 2):174S–185S.

Gowers WR. *A Manual of Diseases of the Nervous System.* 1866.

Henchcliffe C, Schumacher HC, Burgut FT. Recent advances in Parkinson's disease therapy: use of monoamine oxidase inhibitors. *Expert Rev Neurother.* 2005;5(6):811–821.

Katzenschlager R, Evans A, Manson A, et al. Mucuna pruriens in Parkinson's disease: a double blind clinical and pharmacological study. *J Neurol Neurosurg Psychiatry.* 2004;75(12):1672–1627.

Lew MF. Selegiline orally disintegrating tablets for the treatment of Parkinson's disease. *Expert Rev Neurother.* 2005;5(6):705–712.

Lew MF, Pahwa R, Leehey M, Bertoni J, Kricorian G; The Zydis Segeline Study Group. Safety and efficacy of newly formulated selegiline orally disintegrating tablets as an adjunct to levodopa in the management of "off" episodes in patients with Parkinson's disease. *Curr Med Res Opin.* 2007;23(4):741–750.

LeWitt PA, Taylor DC. Protection against Parkinson's disease progression: clinical experience. *Neurotherapeutics.* 2008;5(2):210–225.

Manyam BV, Sanchez-Ramos JR. Traditional and complementary therapies in Parkinson's disease. *Adv Neurol.* 1999;80:565–574.

Olanow CW. The scientific basis for the current treatment of Parkinson's disease. *Annu Rev Med.* 2004;55:41–60.

Olanow CW. Rationale for considering that propargylamines might be neuroprotective in Parkinson's disease. *Neurology.* 2006;66(10 suppl 4):S69–79.

Olanow CW, Schapira AH, Agid Y. Neuroprotection for Parkinson's disease: prospects and promises. *Ann Neurol.* 2003;53(suppl 3): S1–S2.

Rascol O. Monoamine oxidase inhibitors—is it time to up the TEMPO? *Lancet Neurol.* 2003;2(3):142–143.

Schapira A, Bate G, Kirkpatrick P. Rasagiline. *Nat Rev Drug Discov.* 2005;4(8):625–626.

Schapira, AH. Future directions in the treatment of Parkinson's disease. *Mov Disord.* 2007;22(suppl 17):S385–S391.

Slattery DA, Morrow JA, Hudson AL, Hill DR, Nutt DJ, Henry B. Comparison of alterations in c-fos and Egr-1 (zif268) expression throughout the rat brain following acute administration of different classes of antidepressant compounds. *Neuropsychopharmacology.* 2005;30(7):1278–1287.

Suchowersky O, Gronseth G, Perlmutter J, Reich S, Zesiewicz T, Weiner WJ. Practice parameter: neuroprotective strategies and alternative therapies for Parkinson disease (an evidence-based review). Report of the Quality Standards Subcommittee of the American Academy of Neurology. *Neurology.* 2006;66:968–975.

REFERENCES

1. Alves G, Forsaa EB, Pederson KF, Dreetz GM, Larsen JP. Epidemiology of Parkinson's disease. *J Neurol.* 2008;255(suppl 5):18–32.

2. Antoniades CA, Barker RA. The search for biomarkers in Parkinson's disease: a critical review. *Expert Rev Neurother.* 2008;8(12):1841–1852.

3. Chaudhuri KR, Naidu Y. Early Parkinson's disease and non-motor issues. *J Neurol.* 2008;255(suppl 5):33–38.

4. Jankovic J, Aguilar LG. Current approaches to the treatment of Parkinson's disease. *Neuropsychiatr Dis Treat.* 2008;4(4):743–757.

5. Lewitt PA. Levodopa for the treatment of Parkinson's disease. *N Engl J Med.* 2008;359(23):2468–2476.

6. Reichmann H. Initiation of Parkinson's disease treatment. *J Neurol.* 2008;255(suppl 5):57–59.

7. Schapira AH. Neurobiology and treatment of Parkinson's disease. *Trends Pharmacol Sci.* 2008.

8. Sommer DB, Stacy MA. What's in the pipeline for the treatment of Parkinson's disease? *Expert Rev Neurother.* 2008;8(12):1829–1839.

9. Jankovic J, Shoulson I, Weiner WJ. Early-stage Parkinson's disease: to treat or not to treat. *Neurology.* 1994;44(3 suppl 1):S4–S7.

10. Jankovic J. Parkinson's disease therapy: treatment of early and late disease. *Chin Med J* (Eng.). 2001;114(3):227–234.

11. Jankovic J. Parkinson's disease: clinical features and diagnosis. *J Neurol Neurosurg Psychiatry.* 2008;79(4):368–376.

12. Berg D. Marker for a preclinical diagnosis of Parkinson's disease as a basis for neuroprotection. *J Neural Transm Suppl.* 2006;(71):123–132.

13. Kumru HJ, Santamaria J, Tolosa E, Iranzo A. Relation between subtype of Parkinson's disease and REM sleep behavior disorder. *Sleep Med.* 2007;8(7–8):779–783.

14. Manni R, Terzaghi M, Pacchetti C, Nappi G. Sleep disorders in Parkinson's disease: facts and new perspectives. *Neurol Sci.* 2007;28(suppl 1):S1–S5.

15. Marion MH, Qurashi M, Marshal G, Foster O. Is REM sleep behaviour disorder (RBD) a risk factor of dementia in idiopathic Parkinson's disease? *J Neurol.* 2008;255(2):192–196.

16. Braak H, Del Tredici K, Bratzke H, Hamm-Clement J, Snadmann-Keil D, Rub U. Staging of the intracerebral inclusion body pathology associated with idiopathic Parkinson's disease (preclinical and clinical stages). *J Neurol.* 2002;249(suppl 3):III/1–5.

17. Braak H, Del Tredici K, et al. Staging of brain pathology related to sporadic Parkinson's disease. *Neurobiol Aging.* 2003;24(2):197–211.

18. Pirker W, Holler I, Gerschlager W, Asenbaum S, Zettinig G, Brucke T. Measuring the rate of progression of Parkinson's disease over a 5-year period with beta-CIT SPECT. *Mov Disord.* 2003;18(11):1266–1272.

19. Uitti RJ, Baba Y, Szolek ZK, Putzke DJ. Defining the Parkinson's disease phenotype: initial symptoms and baseline characteristics in a clinical cohort. *Parkinsonism Relat Disord.* 2005;11(3):139–145.

20. Braak H, Bohl JR, Muller CM, Rub U, deVos RA, Del Tredia K. Stanley Fahn Lecture 2005: The staging procedure for the inclusion body pathology associated with sporadic Parkinson's disease reconsidered. *Mov Disord.* 2006;21(12):2042–2051.

21. Braak H, Muller CM, Rub U, de Vos RA, Del Tredici K. Pathology associated with sporadic Parkinson's disease—where does it end? *J Neural Transm Suppl.* 2006;(70):89–97.

22. Thomas L. George C. Cotzias 1918–1977. *Trans Assoc Am Physicians.* 1978;91:23–24.

23. Goetz CG. Charcot on Parkinson's disease. *Mov Disord.* 1986;1(1):27–32.

24. Herzberg L. Dr James Parkinson. *Clin Exp Neurol.* 1987;24:221–223.

25. Hagglund JV. Hitler's Parkinson's disease: a videotape illustration. *Mov Disord.* 1992;7(4):383–384.

26. Finger S. *Origins of Neuroscience: The History of Explorations into Brain Function.* New York, NY: Oxford Press; 1994.

27. Kowa H. Writing by James Parkinson and epidemiology [in Japanese]. *Nippon Naika Gakkai Zasshi*. 1994;83(4):524–527.

28. Tanaka J, Fukuda T. Historical background of Parkinson's disease: on cellular degeneration of the substantia nigra [in Japanese]. *Nippon Naika Gakkai Zasshi*. 1994;83(4):528–532.

29. Horowski R, Horowski L, Vogel S, Poewe W, Kielhorn FW. An essay on Wilhelm von Humboldt and the shaking palsy: first comprehensive description of Parkinson's disease by a patient. *Neurology*. 1995;45(3, pt 1):565–568.

30. Yanagisawa N. Historical review of research on functions of basal ganglia. *Eur Neurol*. 1996;36(suppl 1):2–8.

31. Jones JM. Great shakes: famous people with Parkinson disease. *South Med J*. 2004;97(12):1186–1189.

32. Stien R. Shakespeare on parkinsonism. *Mov Disord*. 2005;20(6):768–769.

33. Hornykiewic O. The discovery of dopamine deficiency in the parkinsonian brain. *J Neural Transm Suppl*. 2006;(70):9–15.

34. Zhang ZX, Dong ZH, Román GC. Early descriptions of Parkinson disease in ancient China. *Arch Neurol*. 2006;63(5):782–784.

35. Kempster PA, Hurwitz B, Lees AJ. A new look at James Parkinson's essay on the shaking palsy. *Neurology*. 2007;69(5):482–485.

36. Williams DR. James Parkinson's London. *Mov Disord*. 2007;22(13):1857–1859.

37. Hughes AJ, Ben-Shlomo Y, Daniel SE, Lees AJ. What features improve the accuracy of clinical diagnosis in Parkinson's disease: a clinicopathologic study. *Neurology*. 1992;42(6):1142–1146.

38. Hughes AJ, Daniel SE, Kilford L, Lees AJ. Accuracy of clinical diagnosis of idiopathic Parkinson's disease: a clinico-pathological study of 100 cases. *J Neurol Neurosurg Psychiatry*. 1992;55(3):181–184.

39. Hughes AJ, Daniel SE, Kilford L, Lees AJ. The clinical features of Parkinson's disease in 100 histologically proven cases. *Adv Neurol*. 1993;60:595–599.

40. Klein C. The genetics of Parkinson syndrome [In German]. *Praxis (Bern 1994)*. 2001;90(23):1015–1023.

41. Klein C, Schlossmacher MG. The genetics of Parkinson disease: implications for neurological care. *Nat Clin Pract Neurol*. 2006;2(3):136–146.

42. Bonifati V. Genetics of parkinsonism. *Parkinsonism Relat Disord*. 2007;13(suppl 3):S233–241.

43. Klein C, Lohmann-Hedrich K. Impact of recent genetic findings in Parkinson's disease. *Curr Opin Neurol*. 2007;20(4):453–464.

44. Klein C, Schlossmacher MG. Parkinson disease, 10 years after its genetic revolution: multiple clues to a complex disorder. *Neurology*. 2007;69(22):2093–2104.

45. Wider C, Wszolek ZK. Clinical genetics of Parkinson's disease and related disorders. *Parkinsonism Relat Disord*. 2007;13(suppl 3):S229–S232.

46. Biskup S, Gerlach M, Kupsch A, Reichmann H, Riederer P, Viergge P. Genes associated with Parkinson syndrome. *J Neurol*. 2008;255(suppl 5):8–17.

47. Langston JW, Ballard PA Jr. Parkinson's disease in a chemist working with 1-methyl-4-phenyl-1,2,5,6-tetrahydropyridine. *N Engl J Med.* 1983;309(5):310.

48. Langston JW, Irwin I, Langston EB, Forno LS. 1-Methyl-4-phenylpyridinium ion (MPP+): identification of a metabolite of MPTP, a toxin selective to the substantia nigra. *Neurosci Lett.* 1984;48(1):87–92.

49. Tanner CM, Langston JW. Do environmental toxins cause Parkinson's disease? A critical review. *Neurology.* 1990;40(10 suppl 3):suppl 17–30; discussion 30–31.

50. Tanner CM. Epidemiology of Parkinson's disease. *Neurol Clin.* 1992;10(2):317–329.

51. Tanner CM, Goldman SM. Epidemiology of Parkinson's disease. *Neurol Clin.* 1996;14(2):317–335.

52. Tanner CM, Ottman R, Goldman SM, et al. Parkinson disease in twins: an etiologic study. *JAMA.* 1999;281(4):341–346.

53. Tanner CM, Aston DA. Epidemiology of Parkinson's disease and akinetic syndromes. *Curr Opin Neurol.* 2000;13(4):427–430.

54. Tanner CM, Goldman SM, Aston DA, et al. Smoking and Parkinson's disease in twins. *Neurology.* 2002;58(4):581–588.

55. Tanner CM. (2003). Is the cause of Parkinson's disease environmental or hereditary? Evidence from twin studies. *Adv Neurol.* 2003;91:133–142.

56. Dorsey ER, Constantinescu R, Thompson JP, et al. Projected number of people with Parkinson disease in the most populous nations, 2005 through 2030. *Neurology.* 2007;68(5):384–386.

57. Goren JL, Friedman JH. Yawning as an aura for an L-dopa-induced "on" in Parkinson's disease. *Neurology.* 1998;50(3):823.

58. O'Sullivan JD, Lees AJ, Hughes AJ, et al. Yawning in Parkinson's disease. *Neurology.* 1999;52(2):428.

59. Schiller F. Yawning? *J Hist Neurosci.* 2002;11(4):392–401.

60. Thobois S, Jahanshahi M, Pinto S, Frackowiak R, Limousin-Dowsey P. PET and SPECT functional imaging studies in Parkinsonian syndromes: from the lesion to its consequences. *Neuroimage.* 2004;23(1):1–16.

61. Morrish P. The meaning of negative DAT SPECT and F-Dopa PET scans in patients with clinical Parkinson's disease. *Mov Disord.* 2005;20(1):117; author reply 117–118.

62. Laihinen A, Halsband U. PET imaging of the basal ganglia. *J Physiol Paris.* 2006;99(4–6):406–413.

63. Brooks DJ. Imaging non-dopaminergic function in Parkinson's disease. *Mol Imaging Biol.* 2007;9(4):217–222.

64. Stoessl AJ. Positron emission tomography in premotor Parkinson's disease. *Parkinsonism Relat Disord.* 2007;13(suppl 3):S421–S424.

65. Eshuis SA, Jager PL, et al. Direct comparison of FP-CIT SPECT and F-DOPA PET in patients with Parkinson's disease and healthy controls. *Eur J Nucl Med Mol Imaging.* 2008.

66. Pavese N, Brooks DJ. Imaging neurodegeneration in Parkinson's disease. *Biochim Biophys Acta*. 2008.

67. Curran T, Lang AE. Parkinsonian syndromes associated with hydrocephalus: case reports, a review of the literature, and pathophysiological hypotheses. *Mov Disord*. 1994;9(5):508–520.

68. Duvoisin RC. Differential diagnosis of PSP. *J Neural Transm Suppl*. 1994;42:51–67.

69. Taussig D, Plante-Bordeneuve V. Atypical familial parkinsonian syndromes. Parkinson diseases or specific entities? [in French]. *Presse Med*. 1997;26(6):290–296.

70. Camicioli R. Identification of parkinsonism and Parkinson's disease. *Drugs Today (Barc)*. 2002;38(10):677–686.

71. Tsuchiya K, Ikeda K, et al. Parkinson's disease mimicking senile dementia of the Alzheimer type: a clinicopathological study of four autopsy cases. *Neuropathology*. 2002;22(2):77–84.

72. Lachenmayer L. Differential diagnosis of parkinsonian syndromes: dynamics of time courses are essential. *J Neurol*. 2003; 250(suppl 1):I11–14.

73. Mitra K, Gangopadhaya PK, et al. Parkinsonism plus syndrome—a review. *Neurol India*. 2003;51(2):183–188.

74. Sibon I, Fenelon G, et al. Vascular parkinsonism. *J Neurol*. 2004;251(5):513–524.

75. Tuite PJ, Krawczewski K. Parkinsonism: a review-of-systems approach to diagnosis. *Semin Neurol*. 2007;27(2):113–122.

76. Lubarsky M, Juncos JL. Progressive supranuclear palsy: a current review. *Neurologist*. 2008;14(2):79–88.

77. Tysnes OB, Vilming ST. Atypical parkinsonism [in Norwegian]. *Tidsskr Nor Laegeforen*. 2008;128(18):2077–2080.

78. Caviness JN. Parkinsonism & related disorders. Myoclonus. *Parkinsonism Relat Disord*. 2007;13(suppl 3):S375–S384.

79. Dodel R, Csoti I, et al. Lewy body dementia and Parkinson's disease with dementia. *J Neurol*. 2008;255(suppl 5):39–47.

80. Kurota S. Clinical and pathological findings in dementia with Lewy bodies [in Japanese]. *Seishin Shinkeigaku Zasshi*. 2008;110(7):571–576.

81. Poewe W. When a Parkinson's disease patient starts to hallucinate. *Pract Neurol*. 2008;8(4):238–241.

82. Papp M, Kovacs T. Multiple system atrophy: the beginning of a new era in the history of neurodegenerative diseases [in Hungarian]. *Ideggyogy Sz*. 2006;59(9–10):308–320.

83. Bhidayasiri R, Ling H. Multiple system atrophy. *Neurologist*. 2008;14(4):224–237.

84. Gilman S, Wenning GK, et al. Second consensus statement on the diagnosis of multiple system atrophy. *Neurology*. 2008;71(9):670–676.

85. Stover NP, Walker HC, et al. Corticobasal degeneration. *Handb Clin Neurol*. 2007;84:351–372.

86. Rodriguez RL, Fernandez HH, et al. Pearls in patient selection for deep brain stimulation. *Neurologist.* 2007;13(5):253–260.

87. Dowling J. Deep brain stimulation: current and emerging indications. *Mo Med.* 2008;105(5):424–428.

88. Wick JY, Zanni GR. Essential tremor: symptoms and treatment. *Consult Pharm.* 2008;23(5):364–370, 375–377.

89. Wilms H, Raethjen J. Tremor. Differential diagnosis and treatment [in German]. *Nervenarzt.* 2008;79(8):975–980; quiz 981.

90. Atadzhanov M, Mwaba P. Re: upper limb tremor induced by peripheral nerve injury. *Neurology* .2007;69(13):1381; author reply 1381.

91. Nahab FB, Peckham E, et al. Essential tremor, deceptively simple. *Pract Neurol.* 2007;7(4):222–233.

92. Raethjen J, Deuschl G. Tremor [in German]. *Ther Umsch.* 2007;64(1): 35–40.

93. Telarovic S, Relja M. Tremor—clinical features [in Croatian]. *Lijec Vjesn.* 2007;129(6–7):223–229.

94. Wolters A, Benecke R. Diagnosis and treatment of tremor in Parkinson's disease and essential tremor [in German]. *MMW Fortschr Med.* 2007;149(suppl 2):94–96.

95. Ecroyd H, Carver JA. Unraveling the mysteries of protein folding and misfolding. *IUBMB Life.* 2008;60(12):769–774.

96. Kovacs GG, Alafuzoff I, et al. Mixed brain pathologies in dementia: the BrainNet Europe consortium experience. *Dement Geriatr Cogn Disord.* 2008;26(4):343–350.

97. Critchley P, Langdon N, et al. Domperidone. *Br Med J (Clin Res Ed).* 1985;290(6470):788.

98. Champion MC, Hartnett M, et al. Domperidone, a new dopamine antagonist. *CMAJ.* 1986;135(5):457–461.

99. Parkes JD. Domperidone and Parkinson's disease. *Clin Neuropharmacol.* 1986;9(6):517–532.

100. Micheli F, Gatto E, et al. Domperidone and Parkinson disease [in Spanish]. *Medicina (B Aires).* 1988;48(2):218.

101. Okun MS, Heilman KM, et al. Treatment of pseudobulbar laughter after gamma knife thalamotomy. *Mov Disord.* 2002;17(3):622–624.

102. Okun MS, Raju DV, et al. Pseudobulbar crying induced by stimulation in the region of the subthalamic nucleus. *J Neurol Neurosurg Psychiatry.* 2004;75(6):921–923.

103. Siddiqui MS, Fernandez HH, et al. Inappropriate crying and laughing in Parkinson disease and movement disorders. *World J Biol Psychiatry.* 2008;1–7.

104. Uc EY, Rizzo M, et al. Impaired visual search in drivers with Parkinson's disease. *Ann Neurol.* 2006;60(4):407–413.

105. Uc EY, Rizzo M, et al. Impaired navigation in drivers with Parkinson's disease. *Brain.* 2007;130(pt 9):2433–2440.

106. Biousse V, Skibell BC, et al. Ophthalmologic features of Parkinson's disease. *Neurology.* 2004;62(2):177–180.

107. Gasparoli E, Delibori D, et al. (2002). Clinical predictors in Parkinson's disease. *Neurol Sci.* 2002;23 (suppl 2):S77–S78.

108. Sethi KD. (2002). Clinical aspects of Parkinson disease. *Curr Opin Neurol.* 2002;15(4):457–460.

109. Lyros E, Messinis L, et al. Does motor subtype influence neurocognitive performance in Parkinson's disease without dementia? *Eur J Neurol.* 2008;15(3):262–267.

110. Reijnders JS, Ehrt U, et al. The association between motor subtypes and psychopathology in Parkinson's disease. *Parkinsonism Relat Disord.* 2008.

111. Alexander GE, DeLong MR, et al. Parallel organization of functionally segregated circuits linking basal ganglia and cortex. *Annu Rev Neurosci.* 1986;9:357–381.

112. Alexander GE, Crutcher MD, et al. Basal ganglia-thalamocortical circuits: parallel substrates for motor, oculomotor, "prefrontal" and "limbic" functions." *Prog Brain Res.* 1990;85:119–146.

113. Beyer K, Ariza A. Protein aggregation mechanisms in synucleinopathies: commonalities and differences. *J Neuropathol Exp Neurol.* 2007;66(11):965–974.

114. Di Napoli M, Shah IM, et al. Molecular pathways and genetic aspects of Parkinson's disease: from bench to bedside. *Expert Rev Neurother.* 2007;7(12):1693–1729.

115. Luo W, Wang Y, et al. Protease-activated receptors in the brain: receptor expression, activation, and functions in neurodegeneration and neuroprotection. *Brain Res Rev.* 2007;56(2):331–345.

116. Schulz, JB. Mechanisms of neurodegeneration in idiopathic Parkinson's disease. *Parkinsonism Relat Disord.* 2007;13(suppl 3):S306–S308.

117. Kahle, PJ. Alpha-synucleinopathy models and human neuropathology: similarities and differences. *Acta Neuropathol.* 2008;115(1):87–95.

118. Le W, Chen S, et al. Etiopathogenesis of Parkinson disease: a new beginning? *Neuroscientist.* 2008;

119. Moore DJ. Dawson TM. Value of genetic models in understanding the cause and mechanisms of Parkinson's disease. *Curr Neurol Neurosci Rep.* 2008;8(4):288–296.

120. Onyango IG. Mitochondrial dysfunction and oxidative stress in Parkinson's disease. *Neurochem Res.* 2008;33(3):589–597.

121. Rogers J. The inflammatory response in Alzheimer's disease. *J Periodontol.* 2008;79(8 suppl):1535–1543.

122. Sayre LM, Perry G, et al. Oxidative stress and neurotoxicity. *Chem Res Toxicol.* 2008;21(1):172–188.

123. Waxman EA, Giasson BI. Molecular mechanisms of alpha-synuclein neurodegeneration. *Biochim Biophys Acta.* 2008.

124. Miodrag A, Das TK, et al. Normal pressure hydrocephalus presenting as Parkinson's syndrome. *Postgrad Med J.* 1987;63(736):113–115.
125. Munakata S, Nagumo K, et al. A case of parkinsonian syndrome caused by normal pressure hydrocephalus accompanied by the cauda equina neurinoma [in Japanese]. *Rinsho Shinkeigaku.* 2002;42(2):131–135.
126. Factora R, Luciano M. When to consider normal pressure hydrocephalus in the patient with gait disturbance. *Geriatrics.* 2008;63(2):32–37.
127. Chou KL, Okun MS, Fernandez HH, Breslow D, Friedman JL. (2007). Five frequently asked questions about hospitalization for patients with Parkinson disease. *The Parkinson Report.* 2007;XVIII(3):7–12.

I have been having all the signs of early-onset Parkinson's disease since the beginning of the fall. It started out with stiffness in my neck, then tremors of my hand, my handwriting became very tiny, and most symptoms occurred on my right side and a little on my left. I have been reading a book and I have all of the early signs of Parkinson's disease listed in the book along with tremors, rigidity, slowness, small handwriting, change in walking, and problems with balance with some falling.

Can someone give me some kind of guidance about living with Parkinson's? I just don't believe this is all due to stress. I feel like there is no hope left. Your help is greatly appreciated.

CHAPTER 2

Adjusting to Life With Parkinson's Disease

Can I still hold a job even though I have PD?

One of the most common questions asked by patients is whether they can remain gainfully employed with their PD. This question is complex, and the answer will heavily depend upon the individual and the individual's symptoms and circumstances. At the time of diagnosis we usually discourage discontinuation or quitting of the job. Prior to a final decision on employment we prefer that employment status be objectively evaluated and that optimization of medications be completed and multi/interdisciplinary interventions be instituted. Many patients will transform from stiff, shaky, depressed, and scared into optimistic and relatively normal—and they will not want to give up their jobs.

The ability to function in the workplace will depend heavily on the type of job that a PD patient may be attempting to hold down. Jobs that require high stress, long hours, and little chance for meals or regular medication dosing may prove difficult for the PD patient.

We recommend for PD patients who wish to continue their employment to curb their hours, reduce their stress, and to religiously take medications (on a strict schedule), even when at work. In addition, exercise should be considered like a drug for PD, and although working, it is encouraged to maintain a daily exercise regimen.

If the situation unfolds that despite maximal medical and multi/interdisciplinary management, the symptoms of PD impact work performance then it may be time to consider retirement or disability. We always advise caution in retiring too soon, as many patients derive more pleasure and more of a sense of purpose from their work than they may realize (and only appreciate once retiring)!

What should be recorded in my chart at each visit to protect me legally and prepare me for potential disability?

One cautionary note about disability is that every examination is recorded in the chart, and when you apply for disability these records will be independently requested. Therefore if you have a high-skill job such as a surgeon, or air traffic controller, you should be sure a conversation is documented at each visit as to whether your doctor believes you can safely continue to work in the same capacity (you will need to remind your doctor to add this statement at each visit). Such statements will protect you whether you want to keep working or retire with disability.

Do certain jobs (occupations) put one at risk for the development of PD?

There have been many questionnaire and survey types of studies that have examined the connection between doing certain types of jobs and the development of PD. There has been a tremendous amount of controversy surrounding this area of research, especially with regard to welders. The jury is not completely in, and studies have been conflicting, but there are several occupations that may potentially be associated with PD. In a study by Goldman and Tanner (1), the medical records of 2249 consecutive patients from three centers were reviewed for the primary life-time occupation.

Physicians/dentists, farmers, and teachers were significantly more common than expected among PD patients, as were lawyers, scientists, and persons with religion-related jobs. Computer programmers had a younger age at PD diagnosis; risk of diagnosis at or before the age of 50 was greater in computer programmers and technicians. They concluded that health care, teaching, and farming were common occupations in PD patients, but welders were not overrepresented in their sample (1).

There is controversy in this area, and larger studies that are more careful are needed, as there have been conflicting results. One study revealed a decreased risk for transport- and communications-related jobs (2), and another revealed that those with high physical activity jobs also had a lower risk (3). Another interesting but unconfirmed finding was that those with higher education and physicians may have had a higher risk, although one must be careful in interpretation of these findings as these groups are more likely to present to specialty clinics (3).

Most groups agree that pesticides increase the risk, as does manganese exposure (common in minors) and rotenone exposure, but there remains controversy over welders and agent orange (1–9).

Do I have to tell my employer anything about having PD?

Laws about informing your employer about medical illnesses vary from state to state and country to country, so it is important that you review the regulations in your region. In general, your health information is protected by the Health Information Privacy Act (HIPPA) and the decision to inform your employer and/or your coworkers is a personal one. If your PD symptoms may impact your productivity or efficiency, or if you are in a job of responsibility that may affect the safety of others (eg, heavy machinery operator), you may need to discuss your situation with your doctor and maybe even your employer to ensure your safety and the safety of your coworkers. If this issue is of major concern to you, you should be sure that at each visit your doctor records in the chart a recommendation based on your history and your examination as to your fitness to safely continue in your current work capacity. If a legal suit is brought against you these notes will be requested, and the documentation will protect you, so long as you follow your physician's recommendation.

How will PD affect my sex life?

The most important thing to keep in mind is that in regular, garden variety, PD (meaning not MSA, PSP, or parkinsonism), many of the problems with sexual dysfunction will present in a similar fashion to those that may be encountered with normal aging and other comorbidities (eg, diabetes, etc.). Patients with multiple system atrophy and other forms of parkinsonism have a much more severe and early sexual dysfunction, when compared to regular PD.

PD patients have degeneration within the autonomic nervous system, and this is what usually leads to much of the sexual dysfunction. However, the degeneration in nonmotor areas of the brain can lead to mood syndromes that can also be associated with decreased libido (desire) and sexual problems (10).

A loss of libido is common in PD, and recent studies have shown that it is strongly associated with depressive symptoms, which are commonly encountered in PD (11). It is therefore critical that depressive symptoms and mood disorders be aggressively pursued and treated. Loss of libido as well as sexual dysfunction can occur both in men and in women with PD.

Erectile dysfunction may occur later in the course of PD. It is important that when erectile dysfunction is encountered a full urological workup should be performed. In many cases, other potential causes for erectile dysfunction will be uncovered (eg, diabetes, depression). Depending on the underlying cause there may be many treatments including pills (eg, Cialis, Viagra, etc.), creams, and also the possibility of injections or even implants (12–14).

Finally, sexual dysfunction such as delayed orgasm can occur in both men and women with PD and commonly results from medication interactions (eg, antidepressant medications). These cases usually require an individualized approach with medications and timing of medications individualized on a case-by-case basis.

Testosterone levels have been discovered to be low in male PWPs; however, the relationship to libido or sexual dysfunction is currently unknown (15,16).

Most patients with PD will have normal or near normal sexual experiences, but if there are any issues, they should be discussed at regular appointments. Be sure not to be too embarrassed to breach the subject of sexuality with your doctor and multi/interdisciplinary team. If you are too embarrassed, simply place this issue on a list of problems you would like addressed by your physician and hand it to your doctor at the beginning of the visit (10,15–26).

Hypersexuality (wanting sex all the time) can also occur because of the PD and/or the parkinsonian medication or DBS surgery. If hypersexuality or other unusual sexually related behaviors emerge (eg, cross-dressing), a review of all current treatments should be undertaken. In many cases dopamine agonists may need to be discontinued, Sinemet adjusted, and/or an antipsychotic added to the regimen (eg, clozaril or seroquel).

Finally, erectile dysfunction within the first year of PD symptoms should prompt a search for diabetes, multiple system atrophy, or another cause of sexual dysfunction.

What sorts of things do I have to worry about when planning for vacations?

Before going on vacation you should let your doctor's office know when and where you are going and for how long. You should leave them a written schedule of your medications and a phone number for the local pharmacy where you are heading, just in case you will require a refill when gone, or your medications are damaged (eg, wet in a rainstorm or washed in a pair of pants), or lost. Be sure you take enough medication with you to cover the duration of your trip. If you take regular trips to a certain region you may ask your doctor to call in a prescription to the local pharmacy in the city where you will be staying so that if needed you can refill an emergency bottle without hassle.

We advise patients to choose a casual stress-free itinerary and to use a global positioning system (GPS) device for both walking and for driving. Many people choose very stressful vacation destinations and set up tight itineraries to try to see everything in the shortest amount of time. We advise against such stringent and stressful itineraries. The less stress, and the more enjoyment, the better the PD symptoms.

Depending on your walking and balance problems be sure you have assistive devices with you or available to you (you may want to prearrange a wheelchair to be available at the hotel or from a local rental agency). Don't overdue walking tours, and try to plan the more rigorous outings for earlier in the day (patients tend to poop out by mid to late afternoon). Remember that in foreign cities and places there may be uneven pavement, and the conditions may not be what you are used to and therefore you must guard against falling. Have a plan in place in case you get sick or require hospitalization (where will you go, who will you call, do you have some over-the-counter allergy or cold medication packed?).

Drink six to eight bottles of water a day, and do everything you can to avoid dehydration. Dehydration in the PD patient may occur at a lower threshold than expected and can lead to dizziness when standing as well as lightheadedness. Dehydrated patients often struggle with gait and balance.

Can I fly in an airplane or visit high altitude destinations like the Colorado Rockies?

PD patients can fly in airplanes and also visit high altitude destinations such as the Colorado Rocky mountain range. Our experience over the years has, however, given us some insight into changes in symptoms that may occur with changes in altitude. We prefer to educate our patients prior to plane rides and also to trips where they may have an extended stay at a high altitude. We have found that a small subset of individuals may experience adverse events. If patients begin to hallucinate or experience behavioral abnormalities, we like to have a plan in place to reduce medications or use seroquel or clozaril to control the changes. Similarly, if medications do not seem to be kicking in, we advise having enough extra medication to increase dosages if necessary. Not all patients will have changes in their PD symptoms with altitude, but for those that do we advise being ready.

The mechanism for changes in PD at high altitude has not been carefully studied. We suspect that in some way the altitude introduces stress into the brain circuits involved in PD (the basal ganglia). This stress can lead to unpredictable changes and symptoms that can occur not only with changes in altitude but also in emotionally stressful scenarios.

Finally, one must consider that in an airplane it may not be the altitude, but rather the cabin pressure that leads to worsening of Parkinson's symptoms (27,28).

What do I do with my medication regimen if I am flying overseas and there is a time change?

Many of our PD patients enjoy traveling overseas for business meetings and vacations. Whenever traveling across the country or across continents there is a significant time change that may affect medication dosing. One strategy we have found effective has been to tell patients to administer their regular doses of medication on a schedule and to pretend as if they are in their original (home) time zone. Patients should continue this regimen until they go to sleep for the night on the plane, or in the hotel once they arrive. Once they awaken they should resume their original medication regimen at the appropriate times, but in their new time zone. In addition, patients should bring with them some extra doses of Sinemet in case they have dose failures during the transition (especially if they awaken from sleep while making the transition).

How many hours of sleep should I be getting each night?

There is no correct answer to this question. Most experts believe that as you age you will require less sleep. In general, 6 to 8 hours of restful sleep is a good rule of thumb. PD patients need to be careful as sleep disorders are common, and the presence of a sleep disorder may erode quality sleep and lead to excessive daytime somnolence. If patients are arising the next day and feel tired or fatigued, there should be a low threshold for obtaining a sleep study. Sleep disorders are commonly associated with PD. Restless legs syndrome, rapid eye movement (REM) sleep behavioral disorder (acting out your dreams), and obstructive sleep apnea (not breathing during brief periods in the night causing subclinical awakenings referred to as hyponeas) are all disorders that when treated can improve sleep quality, as well as the quality of awake time the next day.

Can I play golf and other sports?

Once your medications are optimized and you have initiated a daily exercise regimen, the participation in sports can represent a potentially great opportunity for both stretching and exercise, and also for personal enjoyment. The most important thing is to discuss with your doctor what your potential limitations are based on the symptoms of your PD. It is important that you not try to push yourself beyond your limits and also that you play sports for fun, rather than in an ultracompetitive environment.

How much one can participate in sports is variable from patient to patient and may change over time, but we have many patients who play a daily round of 18 holes of golf. Alternatively, we have some patients who choose to play only nine holes and to play early in the morning (before the heat of the day). Working with your doctor to find a plan that is appropriate for your individual needs is an important part of planning recreation and in living with PD.

Whatever their sport of choice, we strongly encourage our patients to participate in recreation, and to live as full of a life as possible, respecting any physical limitations to maintain the highest levels of safety. Tai chi, meditation, exercise therapy, and other forms of recreation may also have positive symptomatic benefits on PD (29–37).

What about the use of exercise or tandem biking to treat PD symptoms?

Many PD experts have heralded exercise in any form to be like a drug for the treatment of PD. In fact, prior to the advent of levodopa and other pharmacologic approaches for the treatment of this disease many doctors utilized physical therapy, exercise, and motion therapy. There are stories of PWPs living as virtual permanent inpatients (institutionalized) who were put to work folding towels or pushing the chart rack for the doctors on daily rounds. The doctors were not abusing the patient's rights by putting them to work, but rather they had made an important observation that Parkinson's symptoms seemed to improve with motion. Medical science has now begun to catch up with these early observations. It has now been demonstrated that important brain chemicals seem to be upregulated in PD animals (as well as humans) when exposed to a variety of exercise therapies. There has even been a suggestion that exercise will be disease modifying or neuroprotective. Much research remains to be performed in this promising area, but it is clear that exercise will be playing a more important role for PWPs. Dr. Jay Alberts at the Cleveland Clinic has done some important work where he has put PWPs on a tandem bike (a bicycle built for two). The idea is that the non-Parkinson rider can help pace the Parkinson's sufferer, and if regimens can get to large numbers of revolutions pedaled per minute (90 or more), he has documented significant improvement in symptoms.

Should I manage my own finances?

Neurologists refer to this issue as capacity to make financial decisions. Do patients have the capacity to manage their own finances? This is a complex issue that may expand well beyond the PD, as cognitive function in the elderly may be multifactorial and involve medications as well as other dementing processes and comorbidities. We recommend that full neuropsychological testing session be undertaken and a complete neurological examination performed. An MRI of the brain should also be performed and examined. In our experience we have found the best approach is a transparent meeting between the patient and family that includes both the neurologist and neuropsychologist. The findings of all testing can be discussed, as well as the findings on brain imaging. In addition, the family and the patient can communicate about issues and concerns.

There is one unique situation that PD patients and families must remain keenly aware of. Many PD patients both on and off dopaminergic therapy (particularly dopamine agonists) can develop compulsions to spend money or to gamble (especially scratch-off lottery tickets and to slot machines). These cases must be identified and treated appropriately as well as expeditiously, before thousands and sometimes tens of thousands of dollars of savings are unintentionally expended. Sometimes a plan will need to be put into place such as permission from the doctor to spend more than a thousand dollars at a time, or a guardian for the finances.

Can I drive a car or operate an airplane?

Many years ago, bedside physicians and neurologists used to make driving/flying determinations based on a neurological examination. Recent studies on these topics and guidelines by the American Medical Association have advocated moving away from bedside determinations of driving ability. There are now objective tests that can be run at rehabilitation hospitals to determine the potential safety of an individual to operate a motor vehicle. Whenever this issue arises we like to remind patients that the issue is not only one of safety for the PD patient, but also safety for other drivers, pedestrians, children, and animals. It is never pleasant when a driver's license has to be revoked; however, the safety of the community should always come first. There are less objective style evaluations available for flight safety, but in general we believe that the PWP who would like to fly should have excellent skills in all areas of vision, reaction time, and depth perception. We have found that the driving simulators at the rehabilitation settings are helpful for airplane flight evaluations and can be coupled to Federal Aviation Administration rules. The ultimate flying evaluation should, however, be strictly governed by Federal Aviation Administration rules (38,39).

I am very stiff in my back with a lot of pain as well, which can wake me up during the night. When I get up in the morning it is extreme. Once I move around it's better, but I continue having trouble getting out of chairs and continued lower back pain on and off throughout the day. Is my pain related to PD?

It is relatively easy to evaluate for the possibility of lumbar disc (eg, lower back) disease and this is an option to explain your pain. An MRI of the lumbosacral spine can be useful, but remember everyone has some arthritis, so symptoms must correlate with the level of problem identified on the scan and there must be a good neurological examination to accompany any imaging study. If the MRI does not support significant lumbar disc disease (or spinal stenosis), then it may be reasonable to consider PD as a potential cause of the symptom(s). In these cases sometimes taking extra Sinemet or an extra dopamine agonist may relieve the pain. This medication trial may be the most concrete way to separate PD from other pain. A failed medication trial with a normal MRI does not, however, rule out Parkinson's-related pain, and in that case seeing a PD expert may be the next best and appropriate step.

You should be aware that shoulder pain has been reported by Jankovic and colleagues to be a common presenting symptom of PD. In addition, many unnecessary orthopedic surgeries and carpel tunnel releases are done in patients only later to discover that the pain and sensory discomfort were PD related (10,40–45).

Pain was recently reviewed and studied in a movement disorders clinic setting by Beiske and colleagues. They found that "pain was reported by 83% of PD patients. Fifty-three percent of the patients reported one, 24% reported two, and 5% reported three pain types. Musculoskeletal pain was reported by 70%, dystonic pain by 40%, radicular-neuropathic pain by 20%, and central neuropathic pain by 10%. Thirty-four percent were on analgesic medication. Pain was significantly more common in PWPs compared to the general population" (40).

What do I tell my kids to expect regarding my PD?

It is very important to open a line of communication with all of your children and extended relatives regarding your PD. The most helpful thing you can do for them is to get them as much information and, in person, education on the disease as possible. It is helpful if they can attend regular visits to the neurologist and to the multi/interdisciplinary team. Parkinson's is not Alzheimer's disease and patients and families should understand that most sufferers will have a wonderful quality of life for many years, despite having a chronic progressive neurodegenerative syndrome. A family's understanding and support of you may be the most important gift you can receive on your journey.

Children should also be aware that there are a few genetic causes of PD that have been identified and that if they are worried they should visit a genetic counselor. Currently, it should be stressed, however, that a vast minority of patients with PD (<10%) have an identified genetic defect (46–48).

Can PWPs get pregnant?

There is no contraindication to PWPs becoming pregnant. There are, however, few cases available to us in the literature, so we are unsure what the risk of PD medications may be to the unborn fetus. It is therefore very important that you work with your neurologist to flesh out potential risks and benefits and to map out a plan. Reports suggest levodopa has been safe (in a small number of individuals) and that PD symptoms may temporarily worsen during pregnancy.

If you have PD and your spouse wants to get pregnant, this is also a situation that you will be able to work through. You should be aware that when there is a family history of PD there exists a higher risk for transmission of a genetic defect to the unborn child; however, you should also be aware that the vast majority of identified PD cases have no proven genetic basis. It is important your children are fully educated on PD so that the family can map out short- and long-term plans for a successful life together (49–54).

Finally, movement disorders can emerge during pregnancy both in PD patients and in normal patients. If a new movement disorder appears, be sure to consult your physician (eg, chorea or dancelike movements).

Does stress worsen PD?

Whenever you experience strong emotions, you may feel more PD symptoms. Stress, physical fatigue, and even mental fatigue have the propensity to worsen all of the motor and nonmotor features of PD. It is unknown whether this has a long-term detrimental effect on the PD; however, it is widely known that making lifestyle modifications and reducing stress can improve the quality of life. We recommend a balanced lifestyle with reasonable hours (if working), a regular exercise program, a healthy diet, and awareness that reducing stress can improve symptoms.

Is my bent posture PD, osteoporosis, or both?

Both PD and osteoporosis can result in a loss of height, so it is likely multifactorial. Recent studies have shown that osteoporosis is common in both male and female patients with PD and it is treatable. PWPs have a tendency over time to become bent forward. The best thing to do is to be proactive. Meet with your Parkinson's doctor and be sure your dopaminergic drugs are optimized. Start physical therapy, stretching, and exercise and alert your therapist you desire to straighten your posture if possible. Finally, involve either your primary care doctor or an endocrinologist for diagnosis and treatment of your osteoporosis (perhaps with one of many osteoporosis drugs that are now FDA approved) (55–59). Bone mineral density is now widely recognized to be low in PD, and with the increased risk of falls you want your bones to be as strong as possible to avoid fractures.

I am having cancer treatment and would like to know how I should handle my PD?

We like to advise patients with cancer to immediately open a line of communication between the neurologist and the oncologist. In most cases it is important to address the tumor/cancer as aggressively as possible and to manage the PD as a secondary, but very important, issue. There may be worsening of PD during cancer treatment from many causes (the stress of the therapies, infections, side effects of chemotherapy, etc.). It is important in Parkinson's cancer patients to prevent falling, improve nutrition, and to reoptimize Parkinson's drugs (and drug delivery) during cancer therapy, as well as to tailor regimens on a patient-specific basis.

Should PD patients get the shingles/pneumovax vaccine?

If your general doctor believes you can tolerate the vaccination, we have no reason to believe there is any increased risk of side effects in a PD patient. Those elderly individuals (and sometimes younger individuals) will tell you that shingles is a terrible rash that is accompanied by pain, and the pain may persist for weeks and even months after the rash resolves. Although there are no guidelines in PD for the vaccine, it is reasonable to seek the shot from your internist or family doctor. The same recommendation holds for the pneumovax. If your doctor feels you need it, it is generally okay to have it.

REFERENCES

1. Goldman SM, Tanner CM, Olanow CW, Watts RL, Field RD, Langston JW. Occupation and parkinsonism in three movement disorders clinics. *Neurology.* 2005;65(9):1430–1435.

2. Dick S, Semple S, Dick F, Seaton A. Occupational titles as risk factors for Parkinson's disease. *Occup Med (Lond).* 2007;57(1):50–56.
3. Frigerio R, Elbaz A, Sanft KR, et al. Education and occupations preceding Parkinson disease: a population-based case-control study. *Neurology.* 2005;65(10):1575–1583.
4. Tsui JK, Calne DB, Wang Y, Schulzer M, Marion SA. Occupational risk factors in Parkinson's disease. *Can J Public Health.* 1999;90(5):334–337.
5. Kirkey KL, Johnson CC, Ribicki BA, Peterson EL, Kortsha GX, Gorell JM. Occupational categories at risk for Parkinson's disease. *Am J Ind Med.* 2001;39(6):564–571.
6. Park J, Yoo CI, Kim JW, et al. Occupations and Parkinson's disease: a multicenter case-control study in South Korea. *Neurotoxicology.* 2005;26(1):99–105.
7. Edwards TM, Myers JP. Environmental exposures and gene regulation in disease etiology. *Cien Saude Colet.* 2008;13(1):269–281.
8. Hatcher JM, Pennell KD, Miller GW. Parkinson's disease and pesticides: a toxicological perspective. *Trends Pharmacol Sci.* 2008;29(6):322–329.
9. Li X, Sundquist J, Sundquist K, et al. Socioeconomic and occupational groups and Parkinson's disease: a nationwide study based on hospitalizations in Sweden. *Int Arch Occup Environ Health.* 2008;82:235–241.
10. Chaudhuri KR, Martinez-Martin P. Quantitation of non-motor symptoms in Parkinson's disease. *Eur J Neurol.* 2008;15(suppl 2):2–7.
11. Miller KM, Okun MS, Fernandez HF, Jacobson CET, Rodriguez RL, Bowers D. Depression symptoms in movement disorders: comparing Parkinson's disease, dystonia, and essential tremor. *Mov Disord.* 2007;22(5):666–672.
12. Basson R. Sex and idiopathic Parkinson's disease. *Adv Neurol.* 2001; 86: 295–300.
13. Magerkurth C, Schnitzer R, Braune S. Symptoms of autonomic failure in Parkinson's disease: prevalence and impact on daily life. *Clin Auton Res.* 2005;15(2):76–82.
14. Papatsoris AG, Deliveliotis C, Singerb C, Papapetropoulosb S. Erectile dysfunction in Parkinson's disease. *Urology.* 2006;67(3):447–451.
15. Okun MS, McDonald WM, DeLong MR. Refractory nonmotor symptoms in male patients with Parkinson disease due to testosterone deficiency: a common unrecognized comorbidity. *Arch Neurol.* 2002;59(5):807–811.
16. Okun MS, Walter BL, McDonald WM, et al. Beneficial effects of testosterone replacement for the nonmotor symptoms of Parkinson disease. *Arch Neurol.* 2002;59(11):1750–1753.
17. Wermuth L, Stenager E. Sexual problems in young patients with Parkinson's disease. *Acta Neurol Scand.* 1995;91(6):453–455.
18. Beier KM, Luders M, Boxdorfer SA. Sexuality and partnership aspects of Parkinson disease. Results of an empirical study of patients and their partners [in German]. *Fortschr Neurol Psychiatr.* 2000;68(12):564–575.
19. Roane DM, Yu M, Feinberg TE, Rogers JD. Hypersexuality after pallidal surgery in Parkinson disease. *Neuropsychiatry Neuropsychol Behav Neurol.* 2002;15(4):247–251.

20. Adler CH. Nonmotor complications in Parkinson's disease. *Mov Disord.* 2005;20(suppl 11):S23–S29.

21. Ferreri F, Agbokou C, Gauthier S. Recognition and management of neuropsychiatric complications in Parkinson's disease. *CMAJ.* 2006;175(12):1545–1552.

22. Driver-Dunckley ED, Noble BN, Hentz JG, et al. Gambling and increased sexual desire with dopaminergic medications in restless legs syndrome. *Clin Neuropharmacol* 2007;30(5):249–255.

23. Kummer A, Cardoso F, Teixeira AL. Loss of libido in Parkinson's disease. *J Sex Med.* 2008;6:1024–1031.

24. Munhoz RP, Fabiani G, Becker N, Teive HA. Increased frequency and range of sexual behavior in a patient with Parkinson's disease after use of pramipexole: a case report. *J Sex Med.* 2009;6:1177–1180.

25. Rektorova I, Balaz M, Svatova J, et al. Effects of ropinirole on nonmotor symptoms of Parkinson disease: a prospective multicenter study. *Clin Neuropharmacol.* 2008;31(5):261–266.

26. Solimeo S. Sex and gender in older adults' experience of Parkinson's disease. *J Gerontol B Psychol Sci Soc Sci.* 2008;63(1):S42–S48.

27. Brown J. Aircraft cabin pressure and parkinsonian symptoms. *BMJ.* 1994;309(6967):1516.

28. Bagshaw M. Aircraft cabin pressure and parkinsonian symptoms. *BMJ.* 1995;310(6978):533.

29. Pellecchia MT, Grasso A, Biancardi LG, Squillante M, Bonavita V, Barone P. Physical therapy in Parkinson's disease: an open long-term rehabilitation trial. *J Neurol.* 2004;251(5):595–598.

30. Frenkel-Toledo S, Giladi N, Peretz C, Herman T, Gruendlinger L, Hausdorff JM. Treadmill walking as an external pacemaker to improve gait rhythm and stability in Parkinson's disease. *Mov Disord.* 2005;20(9):1109–1114.

31. Venglar M. Case report: Tai Chi and parkinsonism. *Physiother Res Int.* 2005;10(2):116–1121.

32. Rochester L, Jones D, Hetherington V, et al. Gait and gait-related activities and fatigue in Parkinson's disease: what is the relationship? *Disabil Rehabil.* 2006;28(22):1365–1371.

33. Li F, Harmer P, Fisher KJ, Xu J, Fitzgerald K, Vongjaturapat N. Tai Chi-based exercise for older adults with Parkinson's disease: a pilot-program evaluation. *J Aging Phys Act.* 2007;15(2):139–151.

34. Canning CG, Ada L, Woodhouse E. Multiple-task walking training in people with mild to moderate Parkinson's disease: a pilot study. *Clin Rehabil.* 2008;22(3):226–233.

35. Fisher BE, Wu AD, Salem GJ, et al. The effect of exercise training in improving motor performance and corticomotor excitability in people with early Parkinson's disease. *Arch Phys Med Rehabil.* 2008;89(7):1221–1229.

36. Klein PJ. Tai Chi Chuan in the management of Parkinson's disease and Alzheimer's disease. *Med Sport Sci.* 2008;52:173–181.

37. Mak MK, Patla A, Hui-Chan C. Sudden turn during walking is impaired in people with Parkinson's disease. *Exp Brain Res.* 2008;190(1):43–51.

38. Schmutzhard E. Flying fitness of patients with neurologic diseases—aircraft travel and the central nervous system [in German]. *Wien Med Wochenschr.* 2002;152(17–18):466–468.

39. Park RM, Schulte PA. Potential occupational risks for neurodegenerative diseases. *Am J Ind Med.* 2005;48(1):63–77.

40. Beiske AG, Loge JH, Rønningen A, Svensson E. Pain in Parkinson's disease: prevalence and characteristics. *Pain.* 2009;141:173–177.

41. Boivie J. Pain in Parkinson's disease (PD). *Pain.* 2009;141:2–3.

42. Defazio G, Berardelli A, Fabbrini G, et al. Pain as a nonmotor symptom of Parkinson disease: evidence from a case-control study. *Arch Neurol.* 2008;65(9):1191–1194.

43. Silva EG, Viana MA, Quagliato EM. Pain in Parkinson's disease: analysis of 50 cases in a clinic of movement disorders. *Arq Neuropsiquiatr.* 2008;66(1):26–29.

44. Stamey W, Davidson A, Jankovic J. Shoulder pain: a presenting symptom of Parkinson disease. *J Clin Rheumatol.* 2008;14(4):253–254.

45. Williams DR, Lees AJ. How do patients with parkinsonism present? A clinicopathological study. *Intern Med J.* 2008;39:7–12.

46. Pankratz N, Foroud T. Genetics of Parkinson disease. *Genet Med.* 2007;9(12):801–811.

47. Suchowersky O. The genetics of Parkinson disease: to test or not to test. *Can J Neurol Sci.* 2007;34(3):266–267.

48. Healy DG, Wood NW, Schapira AH. Test for LRRK2 mutations in patients with Parkinson's disease. *Pract Neurol.* 2008;8(6):381–385.

49. Routiot T, Lurel S, Denis E, Barbarino-Monnier P. Parkinson's disease and pregnancy: case report and literature review [in French]. *J Gynecol Obstet Biol Reprod (Paris).* 2000;29(5):454–457.

50. Martignoni E, Nappi RE, Citterio A, et al. Parkinson's disease and reproductive life events. *Neurol Sci.* 2002;23(suppl 2):S85–S86.

51. Scott M, Chowdhury M. Pregnancy in Parkinson's disease: unique case report and review of the literature. *Mov Disord.* 2005;20(8):1078–1079.

52. Bordelon YM, Smith M. Movement disorders in pregnancy. *Semin Neurol.* 2007;27(5):467–475.

53. Rubin SM. Parkinson's disease in women. *Dis Mon.* 2007;53(4):206–213.

54. Robottom BJ, Mullins RJ, Shulman LM. Pregnancy in Parkinson's disease: case report and discussion. *Expert Rev Neurother.* 2008;8(12):1799–1805.

55. Cronin H, Casey MC, Inderhaugh J, Bernard Walsh J. Osteoporosis in patients with Parkinson's disease. *J Am Geriatr Soc.* 2006;54(11):1797–1798.

56. Bezza A, Ouzzif Z, Naji H, et al. Prevalence and risk factors of osteoporosis in patients with Parkinson's disease. *Rheumatol Int.* 2008;28(12):1205–1209.

57. Di Monaco M, Vallero F, Di Monaco R, Tappero R, Cavanna A. Type of hip fracture in patients with Parkinson disease is associated with femoral bone mineral density. *Arch Phys Med Rehabil.* 2008;89(12):2297–2301.

58. Fink HA, Kuskowski MA, Taylor BC, et al. Association of Parkinson's disease with accelerated bone loss, fractures and mortality in older men: the Osteoporotic Fractures in Men (MrOS) Study. *Osteoporos Int.* 2008;19(9):1277–1282.

59. Kamanli A, Ardicoglu O, Ozgocmen S, Yoldas TK. Bone mineral density in patients with Parkinson's disease. *Aging Clin Exp Res.* 2008;20(3):277–279.

Although I was diagnosed only a few months ago, I have had tremors in my left arm for almost 3 years. I am noticing that my tremors are worsening and my left arm and leg are starting to spasm. I am so stiff some days and in pain all over (back and neck especially) that I have trouble walking.

My question is this—I have been told by my family doctor that "you're not going to have a lot of trouble with Parkinson's disease" and that Parkinson's progresses very slowly, yet I am having more and more difficulty with balance, pain, stiffness and spasms. Do some people progress more quickly than others? Is there a rule of thumb as to how many months or years before persons with Parkinson's disease see their symptoms getting worse? Do patients with Parkinson's disease plateau for a period of years and then worsen or is it usually very gradual and almost unnoticeable?

God bless you and all the help that you give to patients with Parkinson's disease.

CHAPTER 3

Motor Symptoms

Is "asymmetry" of motor symptoms really important in Parkinson's disease?

As we mentioned in the earlier chapters, the three main motor features of PD are (a) bradykinesia (or slowness of movement), (b) muscular rigidity (or muscle stiffness), and (c) resting tremor (a rhythmic to-and-fro movement of groups of muscle when they are at rest) (1–4). Often, a later motor feature will include walking and balance problems. Indeed, PD is generally an asymmetric condition, meaning symptoms often start on one side of the body, and symptoms are usually worse on the side where the symptoms first appeared. Having said that, one out of five patients suffering from this disorder will not remember that their symptoms first started on a particular side of the body. The side of onset (left or right) does not have an association with a patient's brain hemisphere dominance (ie, it has no relation to being left- or right-handed). Asymmetry is important because most of the other neurodegenerative disorders (with only a few exceptions like cortico-basal-ganglionic degeneration) that mimic PD present in a more symmetric fashion, meaning they equally involve both sides of the body from the onset. However, while this is a helpful rule, it not an absolute one.

Also, the side of involvement may have implications for treatment. When a right-handed man presents with poor coordination and tremor of his right hand, his clinician might treat this differently than the next person with Parkinson's disease (PWP) who is also right-handed but the symptoms are mostly on the left side. The former patient may need quicker attention and a more aggressive treatment plan.

Do motor symptoms really start and stay on one side?

While the motor symptoms start on one side, they do eventually cross over. However, the symptoms usually remain worse on the side where they started throughout the disease course (and this includes the severity of *motor fluctuations* and *dyskinesias*, which we will talk about later in this chapter). The progression of PD is different from patient to patient. Sometimes, the progression is slow, and we barely notice any worsening when we see our patients during their yearly checkup. Sometimes, the progression is rather fast, and we notice a change during their quarterly clinic checkup. But the general rule is that there is a slow, steady progression with crossing over of symptoms to the other side of the body. In fact, if they never cross and they remain on one side year after year, then we start suspecting that our patient may be suffering from a different condition called hemi-body parkinsonism or hemi-parkinsonism syndrome, which is a rare mimicker of PD.

Can you explain what doctors mean by bradykinesia and its implication in PD?

Bradykinesia is the term we use for slowness in initiating movements and in sustaining repetitive movements. Usually, this is also accompanied by a progressive reduction in the speed and amplitude of the repetitive movement. We test these in clinic by making you do repetitive movements as fast and as wide as you can, such as opening and closing your hands, doing rapid pronation and supination of your wrists (like turning a light bulb), asking you to quickly tap your index finger on the thumb, and by making you tap your heel repeatedly as high and as fast as you can. Sometimes, we use the term *hypokinesia*, which simply means "poverty of movement."

Bradykinesia and hypokinesia are extremely important because the majority of the motor symptoms and functional limitations in PD are a direct effect of bradykinesia and hypokinesia (5).

- Loss of arm swing
- Difficulty with walking, a tendency to drag a leg in early disease
- Increasingly small handwriting (micrographia)
- Difficulty with fine hand movements—buttoning, zipping, and cutting food
- Difficulty turning in bed
- Loss of facial expression, often described as a masklike face (hypomimia)
- Hypophonia (when we notice reduced voice volume and modulation)

What about rigidity? How do you test for it?

Rigidity is an involuntary increase in muscle tone. Simply put, it is our medical term for stiffness. It can affect all muscle groups in the body. We use the phrase *lead-pipe rigidity* if the stiffness is smooth and present throughout the range of movement. We use the term *cogwheel rigidity* when it feels ratchety when we perform passive full range of motion of a limb. When tremor is superimposed on stiffness, this cogwheel characteristic can be appreciated by your clinician. But cogwheel rigidity can also occur independent of tremor.

Rigidity is tested by passively moving the arm or leg through normal ranges of movements. Sometimes, the rigidity is very mild and can only be appreciated by activation, ie, by asking you to open and close your left hand while we check your muscle tone on the right side. One of the first signs of PD is loss of arm swing on one side of the body. This may be a manifestation of rigidity. Later on, if uncorrected, it can lead to what is referred to as a frozen shoulder. Therefore, not uncommonly, our patients initially see a rheumatologist or an orthopedic surgeon for the shoulder pain or frozen shoulder, which was actually the first motor sign of PD.

How do you know that my tremor is specific for PD? Lots of other people shake.

You are correct. Several other nonparkinsonian conditions have shaking as a prominent feature. We define tremor as an involuntary rhythmic back and forth movement of any body part (such as the fingers, hands, legs, lips, chin, head, etc). Rest tremor is the one that is typical for PD. It is shaking that occurs when the body part is relaxed (eg, when your arms and hands are resting on your lap while you are seated). This is the strongest clue that tells us that your tremor is most likely parkinsonian. However, other types of tremors also occur in PD. Postural tremor occurs when a posture is sustained (eg, when your arm is outstretched). Action tremor occurs when performing a task (such as when you reach for a cup or write a sentence while holding a pen).

My doctor told me that my tremor should stop when I am sleeping; Is this true?

Tremor is the most widely known feature of PD. It usually disappears during deep sleep. However, contrary to our old notion, we now know that our patients are not lying or exaggerating when they tell us that they shake even when they are asleep. Indeed, tremors can persist, but only during the *light stages* of sleep.

What other clues point toward a parkinsonian tremor?

Tremor is the presenting symptom of PD in 40% to 70% of cases, and between 68% and 100% of PWPs will have rest tremor at some point during the course of their illness. However, 10% to 20% do not develop tremor (5). Classically, the tremor is at rest, at a frequency of four to six beats per second, but the tremor can also occur at other frequencies. Often, tremors start in one hand and arm and then progresses to the leg before spreading to the other side of the body. Chin, jaw, and eyelid tremor can also be seen in PD, but tremor of the whole head is much less common. Tremor of PD tends to increase with stress and anxiety, but this is not specific and can be seen in many other types of tremor.

On a positive note, when tremor predominates the clinical presentation (what we term as tremor-dominant PD), this usually indicates a slower progression of the illness.

Why is postural instability sometimes included as a core motor symptom and sometimes not?

Postural instability refers to poor balance and unsteadiness. It can and often does lead to falls. We examine postural instability using the "pull test" (when we stand behind you and pull you back with a sharp tug on your shoulders). Patients with an adequate balance reflex will be able to correct themselves by stepping backward to keep from falling. In advanced stages of PD, this natural correction can be lost and patients can fall backwards if unsupported.

The reason this is sometimes left out as a main feature of PD is that it usually occurs much later in the illness. In fact, when it appears very early on and results in falls within the first year of onset of symptoms, we start considering other parkinsonian disorders such as *progressive supranuclear palsy* (mentioned in Chapter 1). In addition, another reason this feature is sometimes left out is that it is the *least specific* of the parkinsonian motor symptoms. Loss of balance and poor walking can be a result of numerous other conditions unrelated to PD such as neuropathy, arthritis, pinched nerves, foot problems, and so on.

Do all the main motor features respond to treatment in a similar manner?

We always tell our patients that of the four (if you include postural instability) major features of PD, two of them respond well to treatment, one is universally treatment-resistant, and one responds unpredictably. Bradykinesia and rigidity are the two most responsive motor symptoms of PD. Therefore, these two symptoms are a good gauge to determine the degree of treatment response when adjusting medications. In fact, if we do not notice an appreciable improvement in bradykinesia and rigidity, we may start doubting the diagnosis of PD.

Postural instability usually *does not* respond to any pharmacological treatment. Sometimes, if the difficulty in walking and the falls are contributed to by stiffness and slowness, it may seem that they respond to medications. However, this is perhaps because of the effect of the medication on bradykinesia and rigidity, and not necessarily on the postural instability per se. Physical therapy and utilizing the safest walking aid (canes, walkers, etc.) may be the best treatment to counteract this difficult symptom.

We call tremor the moody one. It can be a difficult symptom to treat. About half of our patients notice a treatment response with improvement in tremor, but tremor is seldom completely abolished. The other half will not significantly respond to any pharmacological treatment. However, almost all PWPs will respond to deep brain stimulation (DBS) surgery, so when these tremors are bothersome or incapacitating, we consider this treatment. Fortunately, for the majority of patients tremor is associated with a cosmetic or a social disability rather than a significant source of *functional* disability. It is important to differentiate treatment response to the different motor symptoms of PD, as sometimes patients can be troubled by the persistence of tremor despite therapy and may report that the treatment is not working—mainly because tremor persists, even though bradykinesia has improved.

What are motor complications in PD? How do they develop?

Advancing PD may be accompanied by the onset of new motor and non-motor features that do not improve in response to levodopa, resulting in reduced quality of life and the need for medication changes. Often, the chronic use of levodopa is associated with the development of medication-related side effects such as motor fluctuations and dyskinesias that complicate treatment and limit the benefits of levodopa in up to 40% to 90% of patients within 5 to 10 years of treatment initiation (Table 3.1) (3,6,7).

The duration of motor response to levodopa is in large part a function of disease severity. In early PD, the treatment response to a single levodopa dose is constant and long lasting (greater than four hours) despite levodopa's relatively short half-life (60–90 minutes) (3). Half-life is the amount of time that it takes a drug to lose half of its pharmacological activity. Early in the disease, the effect of levodopa seems to last longer than its half-life because there are still enough dopaminergic cells that are able to store and save levodopa for later use. With advancing disease, patients begin to experience a

Table 3.1 Motor Complications of Levodopa Therapy

Motor fluctuations
   End of dose (wearing off)
   Unpredictable motor fluctuations (on-off phenomenon)
   Dose failures
   Freezing episodes
Dyskinesias
   Peak dose dyskinesias
   Diphasic dyskinesias
   Dystonia

Source: Ref. 3.

wearing-off effect, where the duration of effect of a dose of levodopa now slowly mimics its true half-life and is reduced to less than four hours. This effect may be because there are now fewer surviving dopaminergic neurons that act as storage cabinets of levodopa for later use (5).

Over time, the benefits of single doses of levodopa become progressively shorter, with symptoms developing more quickly and before the next administered dose. Patients may begin to experience rapid and unpredictable fluctuations between "on" and "off" periods, known as the on-off phenomenon (3). These motor complications are characterized by the resurgence of symptoms such as tremor, bradykinesia, or freezing (the off state) after a few hours of response to levodopa administration (the on state) (8).

What are dyskinesias?

Dyskinesias are abnormal, involuntary movements that occur in response to repeated dopamine-replacement therapy (3,9). Sometimes, they can be very disabling. These motor complications are typically choreiform. *Chorea* comes from the Greek word meaning "to dance," so the dyskinesias look similar to dancelike, constant writhing, or wriggling movements of the arms, legs, trunk, and sometimes even facial muscles. However, dyskinesias can also be dystonic (prolonged twisting of body parts), or myoclonic (rapid and random twitching of isolated muscle groups) or other movement disorders, and can become progressively more severe with increasing duration of treatment (3,9). Sometimes, with advancing disease, it becomes increasingly difficult to find a dose of levodopa that provides symptom relief while avoiding dyskinesia.

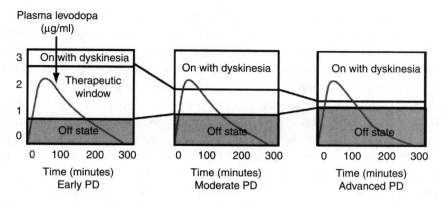

Figure 3.1 Effect of disease progression on levodopa therapeutic window and the progression of motor complications. (From Ref. 10, with permission.)

Motor complications can have a significant negative impact on a patient's quality of life. Dyskinesias that progress from mild to extreme may not allow the patient to rest and may be accompanied by walking problems due to flailing movements. They may be so severely disabling that the clinical benefits of dopaminergic therapy are negated (1).

Figure 3.1 shows the progression of motor complications. During the early stages of PD, treatment is commonly uncomplicated. With disease progression, there is the eventual appearance of motor fluctuations and dyskinesias, sometimes making the disease progress from a nondisabling to a disabling stage.

Does everyone get these motor complications?

Motor complications are more common with earlier use and higher doses of levodopa and can pose a particular problem in patients with early-onset PD (those who develop the disease before 50 years of age). The complications are less likely to occur when the disease onset is after 70 years of age (3). The longer a patient is treated for PD, the higher the likelihood of developing these motor fluctuations. While most patients will still eventually develop some form of motor complications, fortunately, we now have a better understanding of these phenomena and are able to delay them, control them, or in some lucky cases, prevent them all together.

How do I know that I am, in fact, wearing off?

Wearing off is the most common and usually the earliest motor fluctuation that a person with PD may experience. With wearing off, there is decreased benefit from levodopa after each dose (less than usual four hours), and patients may complain that the effect of the drug "wears off too early." As described earlier, drug benefit early in the disease is gradual and predictable, but as the disease advances drug benefit may disappear unpredictably, and even suddenly (also termed "sudden off"). When an *off period* sets in, tremors, bradykinesia, and rigidity begin to reappear before the next dose is due. In addition, wearing off symptoms may include nonmotor symptoms such as *autonomic* (flushing, sweating, lightheadedness), *psychiatric* (depression, anxiety, panic), *cognitive* (bradyphrenia, our term for slowness in thinking), and *sensory phenomena* (abdominal, back, or limb pain; pins and needles sensation; and fatigue). While your spouse and even your doctor can readily appreciate the motor symptoms of wearing off (as they can readily see your tremor reemerging or your walking slowing down), you may need to be honest and let them know if you think you are experiencing some of the nonmotor symptoms. It is important to distinguish whether these nonmotor symptoms are part of an off spell because if they are truly part of an off spell they are treated differently. When part of wearing off, they often respond to strategies that prolong the action of levodopa, instead of the typical treatments for depression, anxiety, pain, and so on.

What is an "off-period dystonia"?

Dystonia occurs when two muscle groups that are supposed to complement each other (meaning, when one group is contracting, the other group should be relaxing, so the result is a smooth movement) are instead fighting each other and are simultaneously contracting. The result is a prolonged and often times sustained twisting or abnormal posturing of that body part. The tricky part about dystonia is that it can occur at any point during the life cycle of a drug response. Dystonia can occur as the medication starts taking effect, at the peak benefit of the medication, as the medication effect starts to decline, and finally at the conclusion or bottom of the off spell. When dystonia appears during the off spell, this is what we call off-period dystonia. A common occurrence of this phenomenon is in the early morning before taking the first dose of medication (because of the long gap between the last dose the night before and the first dose the next day), but it may also occur between doses throughout the day. Foot cramps and toes curling are the most common manifestation of this condition. Dystonic posturing of the arms and/or legs may also occur. Sometimes, it may be a source of significant pain for some patients (eg, severe abdominal pain). The clue that one is dealing with an off-period dystonia is when one experiences relief of dystonia once the PD medication kicks in (and the patient turns on).

Therefore, the timing of the dystonic periods in relation to medication intake and medication effect or decline is one of the most crucial pieces of information you can give your doctor so that he or she can help you in adjusting your PD medication regimen to alleviate this potentially disabling symptom.

What are on-off fluctuations?

The term *on-off fluctuations* refers to unpredictable, sometimes sudden fluctuations, from a treated (or overtreated) state to an undertreated state (characterized by stiffness and slowness) (10). It consists of periods of unpredictable and sometimes severe stiffness and lack of movement, which may last for minutes to hours, and later followed by dyskinesias.

Sometimes, patients get relief from the off spell with an extra dose of levodopa. However, because of the suddenness and unpredictability of its occurrence, medications that work fast, like the injectable apomorphine, are often considered a rescue therapy for these fluctuations. Changing medication intervals, doses, and adding adjunctive medications can also be useful.

What about dose failure? How is this different from wearing off?

Dose failure is indeed distinct from wearing off. In wearing off, one feels that the benefit is slowly declining and falling short of the next dose, while in a dose failure, the medication fails to kick in. The lack of benefit after drug ingestion is what we term as dose failure. It is a complication of long-term drug therapy and is often related to gastrointestinal mechanics (such as delayed emptying or processing of stomach contents, poor drug absorption). When our patients experience dose failure, we make sure that medications are taken alone and not with food. As an example, it is best, when dose failures are encountered, to take medications at least 30 minutes prior to a meal or two hours after a meal. If meal times are unavoidable, it is best to limit protein-rich foods, as the large amino acids from a hearty cheeseburger will compete with levodopa absorption in the small intestines (10). Occasionally, we will order gastric emptying studies to be sure there is not a treatable absorption problem (eg, gastroparesis).

Is freezing also a motor fluctuation?

Yes, freezing can be a motor fluctuation. Freezing occurs when a patient has difficulty initiating gait, walking, or other movements. *Start hesitation* may be the most common form of freezing, but it can occur at any portion of the walking process, such as during turns (what we call turn hesitation). Freezing can occur suddenly and during on and off stages. It may be a source of great disability for patients, limiting mobility and contributing to frequent falls. On freezing can be very difficult to treat. Freezing in the off state may respond to medication optimization.

I experience dyskinesias but not during the peak effect of my medication. Is there something wrong?

No, you are not imagining this, as it can occur. While dyskinesias typically appear at the peak effect of the medication (termed peak-dose dyskinesias), this may not always be the case. One may also experience these as the medication starts taking effect and then again as the medication benefit starts subsiding. This is what we call as diphasic dyskinesia. It is therefore, again very important to note, if you are able, the timing of the dyskinesias in relation to your medication intake and where in the peak and bottom of medication effect they emerge. It will help your clinician greatly in strategizing your treatment. Sometimes diphasic dyskinesias are so severe they will warrant consideration of DBS surgery.

I am not really that much bothered by dyskinesias. Is this common?

The unusual thing about dyskinesias is that, unlike tremors, when they are mild they are often unnoticed by the patient. In fact, some of our patients are surprised when they see themselves in the mirror or on video: "was I really moving that much?" Often, the spouse is more bothered than the patient. In this case, aggressive treatment need not be sought, other than perhaps some assurance and education, as almost all patients would rather be slightly overmedicated (and therefore having mild dyskinesias) than being undermedicated (with reemergence of their tremor, stiffness, and slowness).

REFERENCES

1. Guttman M, Kish S, Furukawa Y. Current concepts in the diagnosis and management of Parkinson's disease. *CMAJ.* 2003;168:293–301.
2. Mayeux R. Epidemiology of neurodegeneration. *Annu Rev Neurosci.* 2003;26:81–104.
3. Olanow CW, Watts RL, Koller WC. An algorithm (decision tree) for the management of Parkinson's disease (2001): treatment guidelines. *Neurology.* 2001;56(Suppl 5):S1–S88.
4. Rao SS, Hofmann LA, Shakil A. Parkinson's disease: diagnosis and treatment. *Am Fam Physician.* 2006;74:2046–2054.

5. Grosset DG, Grosset KA, Okun MS, Fernandez HH. *Clinician's Desk Reference: Parkinson's Disease*. London: Mansion; 2009.

6. Lang AE, Obeso JA. Challenges in Parkinson's disease: restoration of the nigrostriatal dopamine system is not enough. *Lancet Neurol*. 2004;3:309–316.

7. Rascol O, Payoux P, Ory F, Ferriera JJ, Brefel-Courbon C, Montastruc J-L. Limitations of current Parkinson's disease therapy. *Ann Neurol*. 2003;53: S3–S15.

8. Waters CH, Sethi KD, Hauser RA, Molho E, Bertoni JM; and the Zydis® Selegiline Study Group. Zydis® selegiline reduces off time in Parkinson's disease patients with motor fluctuations: a 3-month, randomized, placebo-controlled study. *Mov Disord*. 2004;19:426–432.

9. Brotchie JM. Nondopaminergic mechanisms in levodopa-induced dyskinesia. *Mov Disord*. 2005;20:919–931.

10. Fernandez HH, Rodriguez RL, Skidmore FM, Okun MS. *A Practical Approach to Any Movement Disorder: Diagnosis, Medical and Surgical Management*. New York, NY: Demos; 2007.

My dad, 84 years old, was diagnosed with Parkinson's disease about a year ago. He takes 25/100 of levodopa three times a day. At night he takes 50 mg of quetiapine for sleep disturbances and hallucinations. The quetiapine only helps a little. He also seems nervous and anxious all day. Is there anything else he can take? I am visiting for a few more days and will be taking him to the doctor on Monday.

My 80-year-old mom is his soul caregiver. I'm insisting she get some in-home care for him since she is losing patience with him. He's not the same fun-loving, intelligent man we once knew.

CHAPTER 4

Nonmotor Symptoms

What symptoms are considered nonmotor in PD?

Nonmotor symptoms are features of PD that are not related to movement or motion. Examples of these are thinking problems, sleep disturbances, emotional problems, and so on. Although PD is traditionally thought of as a disorder of *motor* function, the nonmotor symptoms are increasingly being recognized as a significant source of disability and suffering, not only for the patients but also for their caregivers. Nonmotor symptoms can be classified as *intrinsic* (when they are part of the disease process itself) or *iatrogenic* (when they occur, in large part, as a complication or side effect of the treatments used). The most common intrinsic nonmotor symptoms recognized in PWPs are depression, memory and concentration impairment, sleep disorders, and autonomic problems (Table 4.1). Frequent iatrogenic complications include psychosis (meaning, disturbance in thought processing), compulsive, and impulsive behaviors. These symptoms often do not respond to standard dopaminergic therapies. In fact, dopaminergic medications frequently contribute to the occurrence and worsening of these symptoms.

How is sleep affected in PD?

PWPs frequently complain of insomnia (difficulty sleeping) and other sleep problems. Sleep disorders affect up to 98% of patients at some point during their disease (1). Sleep disorders are perhaps the most common nonmotor problem in PD, and one of the few nonmotor symptoms that was actually described by James Parkinson in his original essay, "The Shaking Palsy." The causes of sleep disturbances in PD are often varied. They may arise

Table 4.1 Intrinsic and Iatrogenic Nonmotor Features in Parkinson's Disease

Intrinsic features	Iatrogenic complications
Behavioral features	Impulse control disorders
Depression	Pathological gambling
Anxiety	Excessive spending
Panic attacks	Hypersexuality
Social phobia	Binge eating
Generalized anxiety disorder	Compulsive behaviors
Apathy	Punding (a type of repetitive
Memory and concentration problems	behavior)
Executive dysfunction (*problems*	Compulsive dopaminergic
handling complex tasks)	medication use
Mild cognitive impairment (thinking	Psychosis
problems are still minor)	Hallucinations
Dementia (thinking problems are	Delusions
significant and impair activities of	Illusions
daily life)	Sleep disturbances
Fatigue	Vivid dreams
Sleep disorders	Sleep attacks
Rapid eye movement behavior disorder	Excessive daytime sleepiness
(abnormally acting out a dream causing	Nonmotor symptoms of wearing off
physical harm)	Bradyphrenia (slowness in
Insomnia	thinking)
Excessive daytime sleepiness	Anxiety
Sleep fragmentation	Depression
Restless legs syndrome	Panic attack
Periodic leg movements of sleep	Pain
(jerking at night)	Confusion/delirium/worsened
Autonomic dysfunction	cognition
Constipation	Weight gain and leg swelling
Bladder problems	
Orthostatic hypotension (drop in blood	
pressure when standing)	
Diaphoresis (drenching sweats)	
Sexual dysfunction	
Sensory disorders	
Inner tremor	
Anosmia (loss of sense of smell)	
Pain	
Visual problems	
Seborrheic dermatitis (skin problem	
resulting in greasy, scaly scalp and	
forehead)	
Skeletal abnormalities	
Kyphoscoliosis (exaggerated curvature	
of the spine)	
Chronic low back pain	

Source: Adapted from Ref. 2.

as a primary manifestation of PD or may be a result of medications, motor disturbances (such as difficulty turning in bed), pain, nocturia (meaning, frequent urination at night), cognitive problems, hallucinations, depression, and/or anxiety. PWPs may also be at higher risk for other common causes of sleep disturbances including restless legs syndrome (RLS), sleep apnea, periodic leg movements of sleep (PMLS), and REM behavior disorder (this disorder is discussed later in this chapter).

How do I bring up these sleep problems with my doctor?

Given the number of conditions that can interfere with sleep, a complete history is essential to managing your sleep problems. It is important to determine if you are having difficulty with *sleep initiation* or *sleep maintenance,* as these may have different causes. Other important points to address include changes of your PD symptoms during sleeping and waking hours, and history of thinking problems (including hallucinations), motor disturbances (such as motor fluctuations and dyskinesias), abnormal behaviors (vocalizations during sleep, nightmares, dream enactment, leg movements), and urinary problems at night (2). Often, your spouse or caregiver can also help describe your sleep, particularly if you snore or have lots of movements during your sleep that you may not recall during an appointment. Sometimes, when your doctor discusses appropriate sleep hygiene with you, this issue may also lead to a discussion of a bad sleep habit that could be associated with your sleep difficulties. A *sleep diary,* reflecting the hours of sleep and timing of medication dosages, is helpful. When the specific cause of your sleep problem cannot be determined, an overnight sleep study (called polysomnography) may be particularly useful in determining a diagnosis and directing treatment.

I experience what I can only describe as a creepy, crawly sensation almost every night when I am in bed trying to fall asleep. Is this part of PD or another condition?

You are probably experiencing a condition called RLS. RLS is actually pretty common, affecting close to 10% of the general population. However, the incidence of RLS in PD is even higher. RLS occurs in approximately 20% of the PWP population, which means its incidence in PD is double that of the general population.

A group of scientific experts called the International RLS Group has defined four criteria for the diagnosis of RLS: (a) the desire to move the extremities, (b) motor restlessness, (c) the presence of sensory symptoms mostly or exclusively when the patient is at rest, and (d) the symptoms are worse at night (3). One fascinating aspect of RLS is that every patient describes their nightly experience differently. Some describe their sensation as creepy, crawly (similar to how you described your own symptoms), but others use the words "pins-and-needles sensations," "like a worm crawling under my skin," "severe cramping of my calf muscles," "tightness and squeezing of the legs," "electric shocks running through my legs," and so on. One of the most consistent clues that suggest one is dealing with RLS is that these uncomfortable sensations get better, or completely resolve, with standing and walking (patients are able to "walk it off"), albeit only temporarily. Unfortunately, as soon as the symptoms subside, one returns to bed, only to have the odd and sometimes painful sensation return.

Before initiating any treatment, patients suffering with this problem should be tested for iron deficiency as these symptoms may resolve completely with adequate iron supplementation. The use of certain antidepressants (such as the selective serotonin reuptake inhibitors, [SSRIs] can exacerbate RLS, so make sure you always have a complete list of medications to hand to your doctor during each clinic visit.

A similar condition, Periodic Leg Movements of Sleep (PLMS), is a distinct diagnosis that occurs in up to one-third of PWPs and is characterized by irregular twitches and jerks of the extremities, mainly during the non-REM stage of sleep. Unlike RLS, which can really bother the patient, in PLMS the patient is mostly unaware of this condition as it happens during the deeper stages of sleep. The bed partner is the one who is bothered the most with this condition. RLS and PLMS frequently occur together. RLS can be diagnosed by history alone, but PLMS may require a formal sleep study. The good news is that their treatments are straightforward and many times similar.

> **My wife and I now sleep in separate beds because she accuses me of hitting her, but I do not remember; though sometimes I wake up with a bruise and do not recall where it came from.**

Your symptoms are most consistent with a condition called REM sleep behavior disorder. For brevity, let's call it RBD. RBD in PD is characterized by vigorous (and sometimes injurious) behavior during the *dream* stage (or REM stage) of sleep. It can hurt the patient, but more commonly, the bed partner is the one who is bruised. This usually represents re-enactment of vivid, action-filled, or violent dreams (4). Normally, when one is in the dream state, the eyes move rapidly in different directions (that is why it is also called rapid eye movement, or REM, stage), but the muscles of the entire body are actually limp. But because a PWP is generally stiff, sometimes even during sleep, this usual loss of muscle tone during REM sleep does not occur—which now enables them to "act out" their dream. Interestingly, most men dream of defending their wife from an aggressor (thus often inadvertently hitting their bed partner in the process), while most women dream of running away from an aggressor (thus often falling off the bed in the process). It is a fascinating condition. Fortunately, we can usually treat it with a low dose of benzodiazepine such as clonazepam.

In many cases, RBD precedes the parkinsonian diagnosis, and one-third to one-half of RBD patients eventually develop PD or dementia with Lewy bodies. Therefore, although not absolute, when it appears before any motor symptoms, it can be used as a predictor for some type of parkinsonism in the future.

My husband sleeps all day. Is this a normal part of PD?

Excessive daytime sleepiness affects about one out of five PWPs and is often, but not always, associated with sleep disturbances (1). The reasons for excessive sleepiness in PD are varied and, in addition to sleep disturbances, include the effects of PD on the motor function that may prevent a good night's sleep, depression, and side effects of medications used in PD. For example, dopaminergic treatments at low dosages may be sedating and induce sleep, whereas high dosages may actually cause insomnia and disrupt sleep. PWPs and their caregivers should also be aware that certain medications (particularly the dopamine agonists) may be associated with sudden onset sleep (or what has been popularly termed as sleep attacks) that can lead to motor vehicle accidents (5). Patients need to be aware of this risk when starting these medications. They may want to wait a few weeks before driving alone and do so only with extreme caution. These symptoms almost always resolve after the responsible dopamine agonist medication is discontinued.

Short naps (15–30 minutes) may also be helpful in patients with excessive sleepiness, but they should not be taken too late in the day as they may interfere with night-time sleep. For patients with excessive daytime sleepiness without an identifiable or treatable sleep pathology or other secondary cause, stimulant medications such as modafinil, methylphenidate, caffeine, or dextroamphetamine may be helpful. These medications should not be given too late in the day as they may exacerbate or result in sleep disturbances.

What are the symptoms of autonomic dysfunction in PD?

The pathology of PD has been shown to extend to the autonomic nervous system—the internal system in the body responsible for regulation of blood pressure, thermal control, bladder and bowel function, and so on. Over the course of the illness, more than 90% of patients will experience symptoms of autonomic dysfunction, which often results in a negative impact on quality of life (6). Autonomic symptoms seen in PWPs include orthostatic hypotension (which means lightheadedness when standing quickly from a sitting or lying position), dysfunctional bladder control (which results in urinary frequency and urgency), erectile dysfunction, diaphoresis (our technical term for drenching sweats), and gastrointestinal symptoms. If the autonomic symptoms occur early and are severe, this may give us a clue that we are dealing with a different parkinsonian condition called MSA, a Parkinson-plus syndrome that often has motor symptoms that are less responsive to levodopa and other dopaminergic medications.

Orthostatic hypotension is quite common in PD, affecting 20% to 50% of patients. It is defined as a *drop* of greater than 20 (mm Hg) in the upper number of a blood pressure reading, or a decrease of greater than 10 (mm Hg) in the bottom number of a blood pressure reading within 3 minutes of standing. In a typical blood pressure reading, say, 150/90, the upper number is the *systolic pressure* and the bottom number is the *diastolic pressure*.

When orthostatic hypotension is verified, medications that contribute or exacerbate the condition must first be reduced or eliminated. Sometimes, even patients with a history of hypertension will develop low blood pressure after being diagnosed with PD and may need to have their antihypertensive medications reduced, if not completely eliminated. Dopaminergic medications (particularly the dopamine agonists) may also aggravate orthostatic hypotension. Nonpharmacologic strategies that may improve orthostatic symptoms include increasing fluid intake, increasing salt in the diet, caffeine, and using tight, thigh-high support stockings to prevent pooling of blood below the waist. Purchasing a hospital bed, or raising the head of a normal bed, to 10 to 30 degrees may improve standing blood pressure when performed on a regular basis over several weeks. If needed, pharmacologic agents that raise blood pressure may be used (these will also be described in Chapter 6).

Bladder hyperactivity occurs in the majority of PWPs. Urinary symptoms include urinary frequency during the day or night, urinary urgency, and incontinence (2). It is important to recognize that other factors can contribute to urinary disturbances in the elderly such as an enlarged prostate in men and pelvic floor weakness in women. A complete urological evaluation is essential to make the correct diagnosis and provide proper treatment. Fluid intake should be reduced at night. There are several medications to treat urinary frequency, urgency, and incontinence (discussed in Chapter 5). Most of these drugs should be used cautiously in men with prostate enlargement because of the possibility of a condition called *bladder outlet obstruction* and worsening of thinking and concentration. A bedside commode can be helpful if frequent urination persists, particularly in patients at risk for falls.

Problems related to the gastrointestinal system include *sialorrhea* (or drooling), *dysphagia* (or difficulty swallowing), *poor motility* (or slowed processing of food in the gut), changes in appetite, constipation, and weight loss (2). Drooling is more likely the result of decreased swallowing rather than overproduction of the salivary glands. Unfortunately, the anticholinergic drugs that are often used to relieve excessive drooling can easily cause confusion and worsen cognitive impairment. Therefore, they are not a popular remedy for this condition. Botulinum toxin injections of the salivary and parotid glands have been reported to alleviate drooling in PD (7). Nonpharmacologic strategies include sucking sugar-free candies or chewing sugarless gum.

Factors contributing to constipation include decreased physical activity, diminished intake of food and liquid, reduced force of abdominal muscle contractions, dysfunction of sphincters, and side effects of antiparkinsonian medications (such as anticholinergic drugs). Exercise, muscle conditioning, fiber and medication use all play a role in relieving constipation. Psyllium and stool softeners should be tried first to regulate the bowel movement. If unsuccessful, lactulose can be added. Enemas, laxatives, or disimpaction may occasionally be needed to produce bowel movements.

Impotence and other forms of sexual dysfunction are probably underreported in PD. A thorough physical examination and urological assessment should be undertaken before treatment is initiated, as several potential causes of sexual dysfunction may be present including depression, poor motor control, vascular disease (such as *atherosclerotic disease* that leads to clogging of the arteries that supply blood to the penis), prostate enlargement, metabolic conditions (such as diabetes), medication side effect (such as with antidepressants), and alcohol use. Occasionally, psychotherapy or the addition of levodopa at bedtime may improve symptoms. If not, consultation with a urologist and the use of pharmacologic agents may be considered.

If drenching sweats, especially at night, are part of an off phenomenon due to the long gap between the last dopaminergic dose at night and the first dose the next morning, adding *sustained-release* levodopa (such as Sinemet CR) at bedtime may be considered. Otherwise, propranolol or clonidine may be also considered if PD medication adjustments do not relieve the drenching sweats.

Are behavioral complications common? What should I expect for my wife who has PD?

Neuropsychiatric or behavioral features are experienced by almost all PWPs. It can be the single greatest contributor to a patient's worsening of quality of life (8). Thus, it should be taken seriously as most of these conditions are actually treatable. Unfortunately, because patients think that PD is mainly a disorder of motor control, most do not volunteer these behavioral symptoms to their doctors, thinking it is not part of PD. Neuropsychiatric complications include depression, apathy, anxiety, psychosis, impulse control, and compulsive disorders. Like the other nonmotor symptoms, these behavioral complications are either intrinsic to the disorder (meaning, it is triggered by PD itself) or result from treatment complications. Early recognition and screening for neuropsychiatric features in PD is important for successful treatment. In most cases, a *multidisciplinary approach* utilizing pharmacotherapy (such as using psychotropic medications), cognitive and behavioral therapy, family counseling and education are necessary strategies in successfully treating these challenging complications.

Is depression really part of PD?

Depression in PD is characterized by long periods of sadness or loss of interest and pleasure in almost all activities. The depressed patient feels gloomy, has decreased energy, is constantly fatigued, has poor concentration, difficulty in sleeping, and loss of appetite. They can also be preoccupied with guilt, feelings of worthlessness, and hopelessness. Some may have physical complaints (such as poor sleep, loss of appetite, etc). The clinical appearance of depression in PD often includes slowing of motor functions and may result in worse performance of activities of daily living. Depression is very common and can affect up to 50% of PWPs (9). Fortunately, only a small percentage (less than 20%) of depressed PWPs actually suffer from *major* depression (10). The majority experience minor forms of depression.

While depression can result from frustration and a reaction to Parkinson disability, it is increasingly recognized as an intrinsic feature of the illness. The rate of depression does not vary with disease severity. It may even precede the motor symptoms of PD.

Diagnosing depression in PD can be as simple as asking the patient whether he or she has been feeling sad for some period of time or whether he or she has lost interest in daily activities. However, it can sometimes be challenging as some physical features of depression such as insomnia, weight loss, loss of appetite, and motor slowing are also common features of PD. Occasionally, depression can be a nonmotor manifestation of wearing off.

In fact, depression is often underrecognized. Failure to diagnose and treat depression in PD may result in suboptimal management or ineffective treatment, which can lead to significant disability. The initial approach to the management of depression in PD involves optimizing dopaminergic medication to improve motor symptoms and minimize motor fluctuations. Dopaminergic medications such as levodopa, dopamine agonists, and selegiline also have a mild antidepressant effect. *Cognitive behavioral therapy* and *psychotherapy* are often helpful in enhancing the coping mechanism in the PWP (11). *Family support and counseling* may help improve depression in PWPs. SSRIs are the most well-tolerated and most commonly used medications to treat depression in the elderly, followed by tricyclic antidepressants (TCA), serotonin norepinephrine reuptake inhibitors (SNRIs), monoamine oxidase inhibitors (MAOIs), and even Parkinson's medication that have selective D3 antagonists properties (such as ropinirole and pramipexole). These will be discussed in detail in Chapter 5.

Patients unresponsive or refractory to medications may respond to *electroconvulsive therapy* (ECT) (12). (This therapy is not as bad as it sounds, really. ECT is actually a painless procedure and may even transiently improve motor symptoms of PD. However, it can cause some memory loss.) *Repetitive transcranial magnetic stimulation* (another painless, noninvasive procedure using magnets placed above the head to stimulate areas in the brain) also seems promising and has been recently approved by the FDA for the treatment of depression in the general population (13).

How is apathy different from depression?

Apathy is characterized by "diminished motivation, a lack or absence of feeling, emotion, interest or concern." Technically, it has three components: cognitive (loss of interest in new experiences, lack of concern for one's problems), behavioral (lack of effort and productivity, dependence on others for structuring daily activities) and affective (flattened affect and lack of response to positive and negative events). Thus, there is some overlap with the symptoms of depression. However, while the symptoms of apathy can also be seen in depression, they differ in the sense that depressed patients feel intrinsically blue, or sad. They are very bothered by this condition. While apathetic patients do not feel sad, they are indifferent and they simply don't care. They are not bothered or worried by this condition, rather it is often their spouse who is irritated by their lack of concern or unwillingness to participate in activities. The incidence of apathy in PD is approximately 45% (14). Apathy can therefore be a feature of depression or stand alone as a separate behavioral symptom (15).

Unfortunately, there have been no consistently reported effective treatments for apathy in PD. Antidepressants may be tried, and improvement can be seen usually if apathy is a component of depression. But the best remedy is assurance and education. Caregivers need to be assured that their loved one's "lack of care" does not mean lack of love, or sadness or frustration. Once the spouse is assured and the PWP confirms that this is indeed what he or she is feeling, tension in the household eases up significantly. There is a therapy called *cognitive behavioral therapy* that researchers are currently testing for treatment of apathy.

How is anxiety manifested in PD?

Technically, anxiety is a general psychiatric condition that is subclassified into even more specific anxiety disorders and therefore may be compared to a trunk with several branches. For example, a *panic attack* is a discrete period of sudden onset of intense apprehension, fearfulness, or terror that is associated with feelings of impending doom. During these attacks patients can have physical symptoms such as breathlessness, profuse sweating, restlessness, dizziness, and fear of dying. *Agoraphobia* is anxiety about, or avoidance of, places or situations from which escape might be difficult (or embarrassing). In *specific phobias*, anxiety is provoked by exposure to specific objects or situations, often leading to avoidance behavior, whereas *social phobia* is provoked by exposure to certain types of social or performance situations. *Generalized anxiety disorder* is characterized by several months (at least 6 months to be specific) of persistent anxiety and worry.

Anxiety, phobia, and panic disorder are frequently found in PD (seen in up to 40% in some series) (16). It is common among female patients who have on-off fluctuations, with a tendency to worsen during the off state. Interestingly it is also more common among PWPs who are more affected on their right side (17). It can be seen as a separate entity, or, like apathy, it can also be a symptom of depression. Anxiety may be the result of a psychological reaction to the motor symptoms, as patients may feel uncomfortable about their physical impairment. Moreover, severe anxiety reactions can worsen the motor symptoms in PD, creating a viscous cycle. When anxiety sets in, it can become very difficult to adjust antiparkinsonian medications. Anxious patients often experience side effects from every medication that is attempted. They end up having a long list of "medication failures" due to intolerability or side effects. When a pattern like this is noticed, it is sometimes easier to address the anxiety before making medication adjustments for PD.

There is growing evidence that anxiety is also intrinsic to the disease process rather than a reaction to PD disability. Several studies now show that anxiety in PD, just like depression, is not closely correlated with the severity of motor symptoms and dopaminergic medications (17). Anxiety occurs more in PWPs compared to other diseases of equal disability (eg, rheumatoid arthritis, multiple sclerosis) (18).

The management of anxiety in PWPs may entail adjusting dopaminergic medications by reducing the off state and sustained psychological support (ie, family support, counseling). Benzodiazepines have the fastest onset of action and can relieve anxiety symptoms quickly. Buspirone may in select cases improve anxiety symptoms without the side effects of long-term benzodiazepines. These are discussed in more detail in Chapter 5.

The *internal tremors* that are sometimes experienced by PWPs are often associated with anxiety and respond well to antianxiety agents, especially the benzodiazepines.

How common is it for PWPs to develop psychosis?

Psychosis in PD generally comes in two forms: hallucinations (when patients see or hear or feel things that aren't really there) or delusions (which are fixed false beliefs). When hallucinations occur, they are mostly *visual* (usually these are nonthreatening, and patients mostly see small people or animals, or loved ones who have already died, not interacting with them but doing their own thing) (19–23). Sometimes, they can be threatening, but fortunately this is less common. *Auditory* hallucinations (more commonly seen in schizophrenia) are rare in PD, and if they do occur, they are usually accompanied by visual hallucinations.

Delusions are usually of a common theme, typically of spousal infidelity. Other themes are often paranoid in nature (such as thinking that people are out to steal their belongings, or to harm or place poison on their food, or substitute their Parkinson medications, etc.). Because they are paranoid in nature, they can be more threatening and more immediate action is often necessary, compared to visual hallucinations (19–23). It is not uncommon that patients actually call 9-1-1 or the police to report a burglary or a plot to hurt them.

Unfortunately, psychosis occurs in up to 40% of PWPs (24). In the early stage of psychosis, the patient often still has a clear understanding and retains insight, but this tends to worsen over time and insight may eventually be lost. At later stages, patients may be confused and have *impaired reality testing*; ie, they are unable to distinguish personal, subjective experiences from the reality of the external world. Interestingly, psychosis in PWPs frequently occurs initially in the evening, then it later on spills into the rest of the day.

What triggers psychosis in PD?

Psychosis in PD is believed to be due to long-term use of parkinsonian medications, especially dopaminergic and anticholinergic drugs (19–23,25). However, significant medication exposure is no longer a prerequisite in PD psychosis (26). It was believed for a long time that these medication-induced psychiatric symptoms in PD starts with sleep disturbances accompanied by vivid dreams, then develops into hallucinations and delusions, and ends in delirium. However, this theory is now being challenged (27).

How is psychosis managed?

The urgency of treatment will depend on the type and characteristics of psychosis. Sometimes, when the hallucinations are mild and benign, and insight is retained, it is best that the Parkinson regimen be kept as is. However, when a patient is experiencing more threatening paranoid delusions, then more aggressive treatment is warranted (19–23).

The management of psychosis includes the following:

(1) Ruling out the possible reversible causes (such as infections, metabolic and electrolyte imbalances, sleep disorders).

(2) Decreasing or discontinuing minor antiparkinsonian drugs (with cautious monitoring of motor function). Typically, when a patient is on several antiparkinsonian medications, we peel off one drug at a time, until the psychosis resolves or further peeling is no longer practical because of worsening of Parkinson motor symptoms. We usually eliminate drugs in the following order: anticholinergic drugs, amantadine, selegiline or rasagiline, dopamine agonists, catechol-O-methyltransferase (COMT) inhibitors, and finally levodopa.

(3) Simplifying the PD medication regimen.

(4) Adding a new or second generation antipsychotic (be careful: some antipsychotics can be harmful to PWPs. This is discussed in more detail in Chapter 5).

(5) If psychosis occurs in a PWP with cognitive impairment or dementia, a *cholinesterase inhibitor* (such donepezil, rivastigmine) may be considered.

What are examples of impulsive and compulsive behaviors? Am I at risk for developing these?

An impulse control disorder (ICD) is defined as a failure to resist an impulse, drive, or temptation to perform an act that is harmful to the person performing it or to others that may be exposed to him or her. Manifestations of ICD in PD include pathological gambling, hypersexuality, excessive shopping, and binge eating. Manifestations of compulsive behavior include *punding* (a type of repetitive behavior described later in this chapter) and *compulsive medication use*. Although not exclusively, dopamine agonist use has been the most frequently associated risk factor for the development of ICD. Many factors play a role in developing impulsive and compulsive behavior in PD. Individual susceptibility factors such as male gender and large dose of dopamine agonist, and surprisingly, right-sided onset and early PD onset, may play a role in determining impulsivity in PD. Although not an exact and absolute rule, the higher the dosage of dopaminergic drugs, the greater is the risk of ICD (28).

How common does pathological gambling occur in PD?

Pathological gambling is defined as loss of control to resist gambling as indicated by five or more of the following:

- Preoccupation about gambling, increasing amounts of money gambled
- Repeated unsuccessful attempts to control gambling
- Restlessness or irritability when cutting down
- Using gambling to escape from problems or to relieve depressed mood
- Chasing losses
- Lying to others about gambling
- Performing illegal acts to finance gambling
- Jeopardizing relationships, work, or education
- Relying on others for money

Pathological gambling occurs in 2.6% to 4.4% of all PWPs and increases to 8% in patients taking dopamine agonists (29–34). In our own survey at the University of Florida, we found that about 8% of our patients had predisposition to pathological gambling. Younger patients, men, and those taking dopamine agonists were at greatest risk. They were also more anxious and angrier compared with nongambling PWPs (35,36).

As PWPs are often the last to admit that their gambling habits are getting out of hand, it is important that spouses and caregivers be vigilant of this uncommon but potentially serious complication. We have had patients who have lost their entire retirement savings because of this condition. It is potentially treatable. Discontinuing the offending agent often relieves this abnormal urge to gamble, sometimes almost immediately.

How do I know if I have hypersexuality? I have always enjoyed sex.

Hypersexuality is defined as having sexual thoughts or behaviors that are excessive or a change from usual habits, marked by one of the following: abnormal preoccupation with sexual thoughts, inappropriately or excessively requesting sex from spouse or partner, habitual promiscuity, compulsive masturbation, telephone sex or pornography, paraphilias (using other means of sexual pleasure such as animals). It is often persistent and causes at least one of the following: marked distress, failure to or marked anxiety or distress when attempting to control sexual thoughts or behavior, time consumption, and interference with social or occupational functioning (37). So, the big clue here is that if your hypersexual behavior is affecting your relationship with others (and your partner no longer agrees with you or does not enjoy the exercise anymore), you are probably overdoing it.

Hypersexuality and other sexual deviations can occur in 3% to 8% of patients who are exposed to dopaminergic treatment (37–39). Hypersexuality was described in the early 1970s as a complication of levodopa treatment, long before the availability of dopamine agonists. However, there has been a recent spike since dopamine agonists have been introduced into the market. Several studies have reported an increased risk of hypersexuality among PWPs who are males using dopamine agonists. However, in our survey at the University of Florida, both males and females were susceptible to this phenomenon. Men were more promiscuous though and, not uncommonly, they engaged in Internet pornography, prostitution, or multiple sexual partners, while women engaged more in masturbation and demanded more sex from their husbands. Surprisingly, we did not find an increased incidence of hypersexuality among dopamine agonist users in our own patient population (35).

How common is compulsive shopping in PD?

Compulsive shopping is defined as an abnormal preoccupation with buying or shopping, whether impulses or behavior, that are experienced as irresistible, intrusive, and/or senseless resulting in frequent buying of more than one can afford, items that are not needed, or longer periods of time than intended to, and causes marked distress, is time-consuming, significantly interferes with social or occupational functioning, and results in financial problems. Compulsive spending may occur in 0.4% to 1.5% of PWPs (40).

How do I know that I am eating too much?

Compulsive eating (41) is defined as consumption of a larger amount of food than normal in excess of that necessary to alleviate hunger. *Binge eating* is characterized by loss of control of overeating and eating large amounts of food during discrete periods with three of more of the following:

- Rapid eating, feeling uncomfortably full
- Eating large amounts of food when not hungry
- Eating alone because of embarrassment of amount being eaten
- Feeling disgusted or guilty after overeating
- Marked distress

The prevalence of binge eating in PD is unknown. If anything, the typical PWP usually has weight loss and loss of appetite due to several causes (loss of sense of smell, therefore limiting taste sensation, difficulty eating, difficulty swallowing, depression, etc). Binge eating and carbohydrate craving in PD, however, have been also associated with dopamine agonist use and usually subsides when the offending medication is stopped (41).

What is punding?

Punding is defined as an intense fascination with complex, excessive, repetitive, and often meaningless behaviors. The behaviors can include less complex acts such as shuffling papers, reordering bricks or sorting handbags, but occasionally involves more complex acts (also called hobbyism) like gardening, painting, writing, or excessive computer use (42,43). Punding was initially observed among drug addicts (of amphetamine and cocaine) but has now been described in PD as well. This stereotyped behavior resembles obsessive-compulsive disorder.

How is punding different from obsessive-compulsive disorder?

Unlike obsessive-compulsive disorder (OCD), punding is not associated with anxiety or obsessionality (such as religious, aggressive, sexual, cleaning/washing compulsions). As an example, an OCD patient would constantly wash his hands because of fear of germs or contamination, constantly check locks and the stove because of fear of burglary or fire. The

OCD patient feels anxious, he realizes that what he is doing is excessive, he struggles and tries to stop doing it, yet he still eventually performs the compulsions as the anxiety is too strong to willingly counteract. A punder is simply fascinated by doing the mechanical (often meaningless) task. He would assemble and disassemble flashlights or computers simply because he wants to, not because he fears that there is a microchip or a secret camera hidden inside. We have patients who would sort their jewelry all day, copy cook books over and over, weed the garden excessively, and even relieve themselves in their spot rather than stop whatever they are doing (35,43). It has been linked mostly with high dose of levodopa intake. Its true incidence in PD is unclear.

How much levodopa is too much?

Sometimes, it is difficult to tell. PWPs are often very involved in their own care and are really good negotiators when they want or believe in something. And they can be a persistent bunch. We often see ourselves relying on their spouse or caregiver for objectivity. *Compulsive medication use* (44) is characterized as having a need for increasing dopamine replacement therapy in excess of that required to alleviate motor symptoms; excessive use despite severe behavioral disturbance and drug-induced dyskinesias; and social or occupational impairment (fights, violent behaviors, loss of friends, and marital strain). Compulsive medication use has been reported in approximately 4% of PWPs (44). The duration of disturbance is typically greater than 6 months. Thankfully, compulsive medication use has been mostly associated with high doses of levodopa, and not the other anti-PD medications. Having said that, we often observe that while compulsive medication intake is rare with dopamine agonist use, we find it difficult to convince patients to stop or lower their dopamine agonist dose despite experiencing glaring complications such as the presence of ICDs (that they themselves admit to). They again negotiate and say they will limit their spending or gambling as long as their agonist dose is kept as is. Usually, in our experience this strategy does not work.

REFERENCES

1. Thorpy MJ, Adler CH. Parkinson's disease and sleep. *Neurol Clin.* 2005:23(4):1187–1208.
2. Kluger BM, Fernandez HH. Management of non-motor manifestations of Parkinson's disease. In: Simuni T, Pahwa R, eds. *Parkinson's Disease.* New York, NY: Oxford University Press; 2009:83–94.

3. Garcia-Borreguero D, Odin P, Serrano C. Restless legs syndrome and PD: a review of the evidence for a possible association. *Neurology.* 2003;61(6 suppl 3):S49–S55.

4. Gagnon JF, Postuma RB, Mazza S, Doyon J, Montplaisir J. Rapid-eye-movement sleep behaviour disorder and neurodegenerative diseases. *Lancet Neurol.* 2006;5(5):424–432.

5. Paus S, Brecht HM, Koster J, Seeger G, Klockgether T, Wullner U. Sleep attacks, daytime sleepiness, and dopamine agonists in Parkinson's disease. *Mov Disord.* 2003;18(6):659–667.

6. Dewey RB Jr. Autonomic dysfunction in Parkinson's disease. *Neurol Clin.* 2004;22(suppl 3):S127–S139.

7. Ondo WG, Hunter C, Moore W. A double-blind placebo-controlled trial of botulinum toxin B for sialorrhea in Parkinson's disease. *Neurology.* 2004;62(1):37–40.

8. Weintraub D, Stern MB. Psychiatric complications in Parkinson disease. *Am J Geriatr Psychiatry.* 2005;13(10):844–851.

9. Cummings JL, Masterman DL. Depression in patients with Parkinson's disease. *Int J Geriatr Psychiatry.* 1999;14(9):711–718.

10. Weintraub D, Moburg PJ, Duda JE, Katz IR, Stern MB. Effect of psychiatric and other nonmotor symptoms on disability in Parkinson's disease. *J Am Geriatr Soc.* 2004;52(5):784–788.

11. Dobkin RD, Allen LA, Menza M. Cognitive-behavioral therapy for depression in Parkinson's disease: a pilot study. *Mov Disord.* 2007;22(7):946–952.

12. Moellentine C, Rummans T, Ahlskog JE, et al. Effectiveness of ECT in patients with parkinsonism. J Neuropsychiatry Clin Neurosci. 1998;10(2):187–193.

13. Fregni F, Simon DK, Wu A, Pascual-Leone A. Non-invasive brain stimulation for Parkinson's disease: a systematic review and meta-analysis of the literature. J Neurol Neurosurg Psychiatry. 2005;76(12):1614–1623.

14. Isella V, Melzi P, Grimaldi M, et al. Clinical, neuropsychological, and morphometric correlates of apathy in Parkinson's disease. Mov Disord. 2002;17(2):366–371.

15. Kirsch-Darrow L, Fernandez HF, Marsiske M, Okun MS, Bowers D. 16. Dissociating apathy and depression in Parkinson disease. *Neurology.* 2006;67(1):33–38.

16. Richard IH, Schiffer RB, Kurlan R. Anxiety and Parkinson's disease. *J Neuropsychiatry Clin Neurosci.* 1996;8(4):383–392.

17. Mondolo F, Jahanshahi M, Granà A, Biasutti E, Cacciatori E, Di Benedetto P. Evaluation of anxiety in Parkinson's disease with some commonly used rating scales. *Neurol Sci.* 2007;28(5):270–275.

18. Menza MA, Robertson-Hoffman DE, Bonapace AS. Parkinson's disease and anxiety: comorbidity with depression. *Biol Psychiatry.* 1993;34(7):465–470.

19. Zahodne, L, Fernandez HH. Pathophysiology and treatment of psychosis in Parkinson's disease: a review. *Drugs and Aging.* 2008;25(8):665–682.

20. Zahodne LB, Fernandez HH. Course prognosis and management of psychosis in Parkinson's disease: are current treatments really effective? *CNS Spectr.* 2008;13(3 suppl 4):26–34.

21. Fernandez HH. What we have learned about sleep disorders and psychosis after nearly two centuries of Parkinson's disease. *CNS Spectr.* 2008;13(3 suppl 4):34–35.

22. Fernandez HH, Aarsland D, Fénelon G, et al. Scales to assess psychosis in Parkinson's disease: critique and recommendations. *Mov Disord.* 2008;(4):484–500.

23. Friedman JH, Fernandez HH. Non-motor problems in Parkinson's disease. *Neurology.* 2000;6(1):18–27.

24. Fenelon G, Mahieux F, Huon R, Ziegler M. Hallucinations in Parkinson's disease: prevalence, phenomenology and risk factors. *Brain.* 2000;123(pt 4):733–745.

25. Fenelon G. Psychosis in Parkinson's disease: phenomenology, frequency, risk factors, and current understanding of pathophysiologic mechanisms. *CNS Spectr.* 2008;13(3 suppl 4):18–25.

26. Ravina B, Marder K, Fernandez HH, et al. Diagnostic criteria for psychosis in Parkinson's disease: report of an NINDS, NIMH work group. *Mov Disord.* 2007;22(8):1061–1068.

27. Goetz CG, Pappert EJ, Blasucci LM, et al. Intravenous levodopa in hallucinating Parkinson's disease patients: high-dose challenge does not precipitate hallucinations. *Neurology.* 1998;50(2):515–517.

28. Voon V, Potenza MN, Thomsen T. Medication-related impulse control and repetitive behaviors in Parkinson's disease. *Curr Opin Neurol.* 2007;20(4):484–492.

29. Avanzi M, Baratti M, Cabrini S, Uber E, Brighetti G, Bonfa F. Prevalence of pathological gambling in patients with Parkinson's disease. *Mov Disord.* 2006;21(12):2068–2072.

30. Stamey W, Jankovic J. Impulse control disorders and pathological gambling in patients with Parkinson disease. *Neurologist.* 2008;14(2):89–99.

31. Zand R. Is dopamine agonist therapy associated with developing pathological gambling in Parkinson's disease patients? *Eur Neurol.* 2008;59(3–4):183–186.

32. Driver-Dunkley E, Samanta J, Stacy M. Pathological gambling associated with dopamine agonist therapy in Parkinson's disease. *Neurology.* 2003;61:422–423.

33. Gschwandtner U, Aston J, Renaud S, Fuhr P. Pathologic gambling in patients with Parkinson's disease. *Clin Neuropharmacol.* 2001;24:170–172.

34. Molina JA, Sainz-Artiga JM, Fraile A, et al. Pathologic gambling in Parkinson's disease: a behavioral manifestation of pharmacologic treatment? *Mov Disord.* 2000;15:869–872.

35. Fernandez HH, Nguyen FN, Shapiro MA, Cooper C, Wood MF, Okun MS. Compulsive behaviors II: compulsive behaviors versus impulse control

disorders: a single-center experience from the University of Florida Movement Disorders Center. *Mov Disord.* 2008;(9):1335–1336.

36. Shapiro MA, Okun MS, Chang YL, Munson SK, Jacobson CE IV, Rodriguez RL, Fernandez HH. The 4 "A"s associated with pathological Parkinson gamblers: anxiety, anger, age and agonists. *Neuropsychiatr Dis Treat.* 2007;3(2):1–7.

37. Voon V, Hassan K, Zurowski M, et al. Prevalence of repetitive and reward-seeking behaviors in Parkinson disease. *Neurology.* 2006;67(7):1254–1257.

38. Fernandez HH, Durso R. Clozapine for dopaminergic-induced paraphilias in Parkinson's disease. *Mov Disord.* 1998;13(3):597–598.

39. Shaw P, Blockley A, Clough C, Chaudhuri R, Weeks R, David AS. Hypersexuality and Parkinson's disease. *J Neurol Neurosurg Psychiatry.* 2003;74(6):834.

40. Wolters E, van der Werf YD, van den Heuvel OA. Parkinson's disease-related disorders in the impulsive-compulsive spectrum. *J Neurol.* 2008;255(5 suppl):48–56.

41. Nirenberg MJ, Waters C. Compulsive eating and weight gain related to dopamine agonist use. *Mov Disord.* 2006;21(4):524–529.

42. Evans AH, Katzenschlager R, Paviour D, et al. Punding in Parkinson's disease: its relation to the dopamine dysregulation syndrome. *Mov Disord.* 2004;19(4):397–405.

43. Fernandez HH, Friedman JH. Punding on L-dopa. *Mov Disord.* 1999;14(5):836–838.

44. Pezzella FR, Colosimo C, Vanacore N, et al. Prevalence and clinical features of hedonistic homeostatic dysregulation in Parkinson's disease. *Mov Disord.* 2005;20(1):77–81.

My husband is 74 and was diagnosed with Parkinson's disease in 1993. His medicines have not changed much in the last 4 or 5 years. But now he is experiencing hypersexuality. We recognize this but he denies it. This behavior is so out of character.

About 2 weeks ago, we shared this with his doctor who indicated this is common and reduced his pramipexole dose by half (he is now taking one tablet of 0.25 mg three times per day). Since my husband denies being hypersexual, we have no way of knowing if reducing the pramipexole is helping. Can you give us some guidance?

CHAPTER 5

Pharmacological Approaches to Treatment

I am newly diagnosed with PD. What factors are considered by my doctor when starting me on a medication?

You ask a very important question. Several factors require consideration when initiating symptomatic drug therapy in PD. The choice of pharmacotherapy depends on the patient's age, degree of disability, and cognitive status, as well as the impact of dosing, possible impact on the patient's employment, domestic responsibilities, and lifestyle. Potential drug side effects must also be considered. Thus there are a lot of factors to consider.

The patient's age is an important factor in predicting how well certain medications might be tolerated, as the risk of developing dyskinesia and motor fluctuations, especially with levodopa use, increases with earlier/younger onset PD (most especially those who get it before 50 to 60 years old) (1). Dopamine agonists, which delay the risk of dyskinesia and end-of-dose wearing-off, may be offered as a first-line treatment option for younger patients. However, in older patients (which in our field means greater than 70 years old), the dopamine agonists have a higher risk for producing psychiatric and cognitive side effects. In addition, dopamine agonists have a complicated initial titration schedule before a therapeutic dose can be achieved. They require multiple dosing throughout the day, making the use of these agents challenging for many patients but especially so for patients 70 and older, who may be on several therapies for other conditions. Moreover, the elderly patient is less likely to develop motor fluctuations and dyskinesias compared to the younger patient.

Thus, in the currently published treatment algorithm, it is suggested that for the older patient, levodopa may be a better choice as initial first-line therapy compared to dopamine agonists (2,3).

The good news is that recent data suggest that an alternative option for initial monotherapy for early PWPs is rasagiline, a selective monoamine oxidase type B (MAO-B) inhibitor that offers effective control of symptoms and appears to have a much lower incidence of the dopaminergic side effects seen with dopamine agonists and levodopa (4).

In one large placebo-controlled, multicenter clinical trial, after 5 years of levodopa use and as PD progressed, about 50% of patients who were given levodopa from the onset developed motor complications compared to only 20% of patients who were first started on dopamine agonists for their early symptoms (1,5,6). However, the traditional view that treatment of PD should begin only when symptoms become functionally significant has been challenged by some recent studies suggesting that initiation of treatment at the time of diagnosis results in better clinical outcome later in the course of the disease (7).

The patient's perception of the level of disability and its impact on their lifestyle is also a driver of initial choice of therapy. Patients at the early stage whose major presenting symptom is tremor and who have minimal slowness or stiffness may respond to drugs such as anticholinergic agents or amantadine before their symptoms worsen. Rasagiline, selegiline, dopamine agonists, or levodopa may be added as the disease progresses.

The potential of therapies to produce untoward side effects based upon the patient age and comorbid conditions is another important factor in choosing initial PD therapy (Table 5.1). As mentioned, dopamine agonists are not a good first choice in older patients due to concerns of leg swelling, cognitive impairment, and hallucinations. In patients in whom excessive sleepiness and drowsiness may affect daily activities, dopamine agonist use may also not be appropriate (1,2).

Why are occupation and finances also considered in the choice of treatment? Don't we deserve the best treatment regardless of our jobs and our ability to pay?

A careful clinician usually considers these factors. A young patient who works as a sales executive or a preacher or an actor with even mild tremors may require immediate and even aggressive treatment so as not to jeopardize his or her career. However, an older gentleman who is retired may be able to wait a little longer even if his tremors are actually worse than the younger patient just described. If medications did not have side effects

Table 5.1 Therapies Used for the Treatment of Parkinson's Disease

Drug or drug class	Mechanism of action	Side effects	Specific drugs	Typical daily therapeutic dose range	Typical dose frequency
Anticholinergics	Block acetylcholine receptors	Dry mouth, dry eyes urinary retention, exacerbation of glaucoma and cognitive impairment	Trihexyphenidyl Benziropine Ethopropazine	1–6 mg 1–6 mg 25–100 mg	tid tid tid
Amantadine	Blocks NMDA receptors and acetylcholine receptors and promotes release of dopamine	Cognitive dysfunction peripheral edema and skin rash	Amantadine	50–200 mg, but caution is required with dose escalation in elderly patients or patients with renal insufficiency	bid
L-dopa	Metabolism to dopamine in cells that contain dopadecarboxylase	Nausea, hypotension, hallucinations and psychosis, dystonic and choreiform dyskinesias	L-dopa/carbidopa L-dopa/benserazide Sinemet CR	100–2000 mg/d as condition advances. Sinemet CR has about 25% reduced bioavailability	From tid to every 2h
Dopamine agonists	Directly stimulate dopamine receptors	Nausea, hypotension, hallucinations and psychosis, peripheral edema, pulmonary fibrosis (for ergots), sudden onset of sleep	Bromocriptine Pergolide Ropinitole Pramipexola	15–30 mg 1.5–5.0 mg 6.0–24 mg 1.5–5.0 mg	3–4 times/d tid tid tid
Monoamine oxidase (MAO) inhibitors	Block MAO-B receptors to reduce dopamine metabolism	Nausea, dizziness, sleep disorder and impaired cognition dyskinisia, anorexia, vomitting, weight loss	Selegiline Rasagiline	5–10 mg .5–1.0 mg	Bid Once daily
Catechnol O-methyltransferase (COMT) inhibitors	Block peripheral COMT activity to improve L-dopa pharmacokinetics	L-dopa-related side effect exacerbation, diarrhea, urine discoloration	Entacapone	200 mg with each dose of L-dopa up to 1600 mg/d	With each dose of L-dopa

tid, three times a day; NMDA, N-methyl-D-aspartate; bid, twice a day.
Source: From Guttman M, Kish SJ, Furukawa Y. Current concepts in the diagnosis and management of Parkinson's disease. *CMAJ.* 2003; 168:292–301, with permission.

and had the same cost, this would be less of an issue. Unfortunately, this is not the case. While there are common side effects of all antiparkinsonian medications, there are also specific side effects under each class of drugs.

With regard to finances, unfortunately, not everyone earns the same income, or has the same prescription plan, or has the same amount of savings or investments to pay for their medications. Medications are the single greatest source of expense in PD, and this expense quadruples once the patient starts experiencing motor fluctuations. Moreover, because we have a better options and a greater handle on how to use the various drugs available to us, our patients live longer lives, which means we may also need to pace our expenses. It is no longer inconceivable to think that PWPs can now live their normal lifespan. Brand name drugs can be 5 to 10 times more expensive than their generic counterparts. Yet, most patients will tolerate generic and brand name drugs equally. Only a few patients will have extreme sensitivity and require brand names. By law, generic drugs need to contain the same active ingredients in the same concentration as they place on the label (although it should be noted that generics are often poorly manufactured and may have decreased absorption).

What is amantadine? How is it used?

Originally introduced as an antiviral agent, amantadine is thought to exert its influence on both the "passing" end (termed *presynaptic*) and the "receiving" end (termed *postsynapti*") of the dopaminergic terminals that transport the dopamine to its final destination in the brain (8,9). Several monotherapy trials from the 1970s suggested that amantadine exerted beneficial effects on early symptoms of PD, including tremor and rigidity (9). But its greatest use nowadays is for treatment of dyskinesias (10). Its addition lessens the dyskinesias without the need for lowering levodopa dose. Unfortunately, amantadine's well-known side effects of leg swelling, rash (termed *livedo reticularis*, which is usually a harmless, painless, lace-like reddish rash on the thighs or other parts of the body), and significant psychiatric side effects such as confusion and hallucinations may limit its usefulness.

What are anticholinergic drugs?

Anticholinergic agents were the first widely accepted therapy for the symptomatic treatment of PD (11). Prior to 1969, doctors only had anticholinergic drugs to offer their patients. With increased knowledge of the adverse effects associated with their use and the introduction of levodopa and newer agents that provide better control of motor symptoms, the popularity of anticholinergics for use in PD has taken a big hit. Although their precise mechanism of action remains unknown, the observed exacerbation of parkinsonian symptoms following their discontinuation suggests a clinical benefit.

A systematic review of clinical studies of anticholinergics in the symptomatic management of PD concluded that anticholinergics are more effective than placebo in improving motor function (particularly tremor) with short-term use, but evidence of long-term efficacy is still lacking (11).

While anticholinergics appear to be clinically useful in the treatment of tremor, their efficacy is only moderate and may not cover other (often more important) motor symptoms such as rigidity and bradykinesia. Their use is associated with safety concerns that limit their clinical utility. Anticholinergic side effects include blurred vision, urinary retention, constipation, and dry mouth. In addition, they may significantly interfere with thinking, memory, and concentration, especially in the elderly PWP. Examples of anticholinergic drugs are trihexyphenidyl and benztropine. Thus, while anticholinergic agents are one of the cheapest drugs used in PD, they are not the treatment of choice, except perhaps for young patients with significant but treatment-resistant tremor.

There have been studies suggesting that anticholinergics may adversely affect cognitive function and result in changes in the brain that look like AD. These findings are unconfirmed and only reported in a small number of postmortem brains.

What are MAO-B inhibitors? How do they work?

MAO-B inhibitors are enzymes found predominantly in the brain. Their action is to break dopamine into inactive by-products. Therefore, the enzyme shortens the life span of dopamine in the brain. Under normal circumstances, we have enough dopamine in the brain, and the MAO-B enzymes are actually doing a good thing. They help "clean" and keep the balance and flow of chemicals in the brain. However, in PD, there is lack of dopamine. Dopamine is not being produced in enough quantities, so the PWP needs every ounce of this substance.

MAO-B inhibitors block the MAO-B enzymes and prevent them from working, so there are less of them breaking down the dopamine. The net result is more dopamine staying longer inside the brain. Examples of selective MAO-B inhibitors are selegiline (which also comes in orally disintegrating form) and rasagiline.

Everyone still talks about the DATATOP study. What's the skinny on this?

The effectiveness of the selective MAO-B inhibitor, selegiline, alone and in combination with vitamin E (supposedly a naturally occurring free-radical scavenger) was evaluated in the Deprenyl and Tocopherol Antioxidative Therapy of Parkinsonism (DATATOP) clinical trial initiated in 1987 by the Parkinson Study Group (12–14). DATATOP specifically assessed whether chronic administration of selegiline plus vitamin E in 800 patients with early, untreated PD might diminish oxidative stress, thereby slowing or even stopping disease progression and prolonging the time before levo-dopa therapy is required.

Initially, the DATATOP trial data suggested that selegiline slowed the progression of disability significantly, as measured by the need for levodopa therapy (13). Analysis at 1 year revealed that 176 of 401 (44%) patients in the placebo group but only 97 of 399 (24%) patients in the selegiline group had reached the "primary endpoint" (which in this study was the development of sufficient disability to require levodopa therapy). In fact, selegiline was found to reduce the risk for reaching the primary endpoint to approximately half of that of the placebo group (15). However, these results were later found to be benefits of the selegiline. When the drugs were "washed out," both groups were no longer found to have significant clinical differences (16).

Therefore, as far as we know, based on the DATATOP study, selegiline clearly has a modest symptomatic effect; vitamin E definitely does not slow disease progression in PD, and selegiline most likely does not slow disease progression either. Selegiline is currently FDA approved as an adjunctive treatment to levodopa, especially for patients who are experiencing wearing off.

What is rasagiline? Is it merely a more expensive version of selegiline?

Rasagiline is a new selective MAO-B inhibitor that can be differentiated from selegiline by chemical structure, route of metabolism, metabolites, and its side effect profile. First, selegiline is given twice per day, while rasagiline can be taken once per day. When selegiline is metabolized (or broken down into by-products), its metabolites are amphetamine derivatives. Rasagiline is not broken down into amphetamine metabolites. Therefore, theoretically, rasagiline avoids the risk of the amphetamine stimulant-related side effects, such as hallucinations and sleep disturbance, and cardiovascular instability that have been associated or implicated with selegiline use (17). Because selegiline is available in generic form, while rasagiline is not, rasagiline is clearly more expensive than its older predecessor is.

Rasagiline seems to have a lot of restrictions. Can I trust the drug? What is it really used for?

Rasagiline is actually one of the most well studied medications we have for the treatment of PD symptoms. Rasagiline clinical trials have demonstrated its efficacy and safety both as initial therapy and as adjunct (or "add on") therapy. Rasagiline is FDA approved for use in both early and advanced PD.

Rasagiline as an initial therapy for patients with early PD was evaluated in a phase III, multicenter, double-blind (meaning both the clinician and the patient did not know whether the patient was given the real drug or not), placebo-controlled, 1-year, delayed-start trial called TEMPO [(TVP-1012) in early monotherapy for PD outpatients]. The TEMPO trial examined rasagiline's efficacy as initial therapy in 404 patients with early PD not yet requiring dopaminergic therapy (18,19). The primary outcome measure for the first phase was the change in total Parkinson motor score before and after treatment, comparing rasagiline with placebo. Analysis of the Parkinson motor scores revealed that patients treated with rasagiline had better overall function compared to the placebo group (18).

As for its usefulness as an add-on treatment to levodopa on patients who are experiencing wearing off, two large multicenter studies were performed: Parkinson's Rasagiline: Efficacy and Safety in the Treatment of OFF (PRESTO) and Lasting Effect in Adjunct Therapy With Rasagiline Given Once daily (LARGO) (20,21). Both studies showed significant decreases in daily off time with rasagiline compared with placebo, as well as significant improvements in global impression, activities of daily living Parkinson motor scores.

Do I really need to avoid eating cheese and pepperoni when I take rasagiline? I love pizza!

This food scare came about because historically the earlier MAO inhibitors were nonselective, meaning they blocked both type A and type B enzymes. Only the type B enzymes are generally confined to the brain. The type A enzymes are abundantly distributed throughout the body, especially in the gut. They are good enzymes that guard and block a substance called tyramine from getting absorbed in the gut and entering the blood stream in large quantities. Therefore, once an MAO-type A inhibitor medication is ingested, then the road block to tyramine created by the enzymes becomes lifted giving tyramine a free pass to cross the gut and enter the blood stream. This can result in a severe and abrupt rise in blood pressure (what we call hypertensive crisis). Thus, foods rich in tyramine have been traditionally banned when using a *nonselective* MAO inhibitor because they inhibit the type A enzymes.

The good news is that selegiline and rasagiline are *selective* MAO-B inhibitors. Therefore, at their recommended doses, they do not block the type A enzymes, but block the type B enzymes. Thus in our opinion, it is generally safe to eat any type of food (of course in moderation) whether or not they are rich in tyramine. In fact, during the pivotal trials that led to the FDA approval of rasagiline, we challenged a subset of patients with very high doses of concentrated tyramine while they were on rasagiline. Of course this was performed in the emergency room or intensive care units with all the blood pressure and cardiac monitors hooked up, just in case of a complication. We did not observe any rise in blood pressure or any adverse cardiac changes. In fact, most other drug-regulating bodies in the other parts of the world do not impose this dietary restriction. The Germans, Italians, and Canadians, who probably consume more draft beer, red wine, pepperoni, sausages, and aged cheese in one meal (by the nature of their diet and not by the quantity of food they eat) than Americans would the entire day, do not carry this dietary restriction. So our message is that as long as you eat in moderation, do not worry too much. Bon appétit!

Also, my doctor told me that I cannot take rasagiline because I am on an antidepressant. Is this true?

The combination of rasagiline (or selegiline) and some antidepressants (such as the SSRIs and TCAs) can lead to an uncomfortable and potentially dangerous phenomenon called serotonin syndrome. This syndrome is characterized by confusion, agitation, myoclonus (which are random twitches in different muscle groups), blood pressure, and heart rate changes, to name a few. Therefore, whenever rasagiline or selegiline is prescribed, there is a warning not to combine these with certain antidepressants.

The good news to report is that the chances of developing serotonin syndrome in patients treated with selegiline and an SSRI was found to be exceedingly rare: only 0.24%, with 0.04% experiencing a serious reaction (22). Even better, in the large-scale PRESTO trial with rasagiline, there was no difference in the adverse event rates between rasagiline-treated patients also receiving SSRIs and those not receiving SSRIs. Likewise, in a more recent safety analysis of 316 PWPs who took an antidepressant along with rasagiline, there were no unexpected adverse events or any evidence of serotonin toxicity (23). These patients were on amitriptyline, sertraline, paroxetine, trazodone, and citalopram. Thus, we have some confidence in combining rasagiline with these, but not necessarily all, antidepressants.

What about orally disintegrating Selegiline (Zelepar)? Is this really worth the added expense?

A new selegiline formulation, zydis selegiline (or orally disintegrating selegiline), dissolves on contact with saliva and is absorbed mostly in the buccal region. It does not need to go through the stomach to be absorbed. Because it is absorbed through the blood vessels underneath the tongue and goes directly to the blood stream, it bypasses the gut and the filtration of the liver. Therefore, it results in a higher concentration of selegiline in the blood stream that enters the brain. Because the drug bypasses checkpoints in the liver that break it down into inactive by-products, the amount of amphetamine metabolites are reduced 10-fold using the route of administration (24,25). Of course, these are mostly theoretical advantages. As to whether they translate to clinically meaningful advantages remains to be seen. Having said that, we do know from the pivotal trail on zelepar that led to its FDA approval in the United States that it is a safe and well-tolerated drug, taken only once per day (unlike its older predecessor requiring a twice per day dosage), and lessens the off time of PWPs when taken along with levodopa. It is therefore indicated as an add-on medication to levodopa in advancing PD.

What are dopamine agonists?

Dopamine agonists are a class of drug that exerts its clinical benefits through the direct stimulation of dopamine receptors in the brain. Dopamine agonists are generally placed in two groups: the ergot derivatives (bromocriptine and pergolide) and those that have a nonergot structure (pramipexole, ropinirole, and rotigotine). The ergot-derived dopamine agonists are rarely used nowadays. Bromocriptine has been consistently found to be inferior in efficacy when compared head-to-head with the newer dopamine agonists. Pergolide has been pulled out of the market because of its risk in developing potentially irreversible valvular defects.

Several trials have explored the clinical benefits of dopamine agonists in patients with early PD. Pramipexole was evaluated in a head-to-head trial with levodopa that assessed changes in the Parkinson motor scores as well as occurrences of dopaminergic complications (wearing-off, dyskinesias, and on-off fluctuations) (26). This study found that while pramipexole treatment resulted in significantly less wearing off, dyskinesias, and on-off motor fluctuations (28%) compared with levodopa (51%), pramipexole was not as powerful in relieving PD symptoms as measured by change in the Parkinson motor scores. This is true of every dopamine agonist that compared itself to levodopa: they each had lesser incidence of motor fluctuations and dyskinesias but had inferior Parkinson motor scores compared to levodopa. Thus we know that while levodopa use may result in earlier onset of motor fluctuations, it is still the most efficacious (and one of the cheapest) drug we have to date. In terms of safety and tolerability, significantly more patients taking pramipexole experienced somnolence, hallucinations, and generalized and peripheral edema compared with those in the levodopa group (26). Again, this is a common theme noticed with each dopamine agonist pitted against levodopa: the patients on dopamine agonists experienced more cognitive and behavioral side effects (such as hallucinations), more nausea, lightheadedness, and more sleepiness.

Similarly, a 5-year study of the incidence of dyskinesias in 268 PWPs treated with ropinirole found that early use of ropinirole significantly reduced the risk of dyskinesia (by a factor of almost 3) compared to the patients treated with levodopa, but there was a significant difference in Parkinson motor scores favoring levodopa treatment (27). Likewise, adverse events were greater among the ropinirole patients than among the levodopa patients, with significantly more individuals experiencing hallucinations (17.3% versus 5.6%).

In summary, our trial results and clinical experience suggest that, compared to the efficacy observed with levodopa, the use of dopamine agonists results in less effective relief of motor symptoms and often is associated with more treatment-related side effects, especially in the elderly (nausea, hallucinations, postural hypotension, and drowsiness) (2). However, this should be balanced against data suggesting their use may reduce the risk of motor complications associated with disease progression compared to initial use with levodopa therapy.

What about the rotigotine patch? Are its properties similar to the oral dopamine agonists?

Yes, for the most part. The rotigotine patch is also a nonergot-derived dopamine agonist, like pramipexole and ropinirole, but in patch form. It is replaced one per day. It is approved in the United States for the treatment of early PD but is also used in other countries as an add-on treatment to levodopa. Other than the addition of skin reactions, it has almost exactly the same side effects as its oral counterparts, including nausea, lightheadedness, hallucinations, leg swelling, sleepiness, and even "sleep attacks."

Recently there was a recall in the United States because small snow-flake-looking bodies were precipitating on patches. The problem has been attributed to temperature, and it is thought that by refrigerating the patches this may solve the quality issue. We await the FDA's reexamination of rotigotine.

What about levodopa? Is it really the best thing that ever happened to PWPs or should we avoid it like the plague?

It is with no exaggeration when we say that levodopa revolutionized the treatment of PD and remains the most efficacious symptomatic treatment for the motor features. It effectively alleviates bradykinesia, rigidity, and, in some patients, tremor. Its benefits lead to prolonged functional independence and reduced functional impairments and disability for most patients in the moderate to advanced stages of the disease, and it definitely increases longevity.

However, the downside of early initiation of levodopa therapy is that in approximately 40% to 50% of patients whose disease is progressing and who were initially treated with levodopa, motor complications such as dyskinesia, wearing-off, and on-off fluctuations begin to emerge after about 4 to 6 years. The complications of prolonged use and other side effects of levodopa, including nausea, vomiting, and orthostatic hypotension, limit the use of levodopa in early PD and have contributed to the traditional clinical practice, for younger patients (younger than 65–70 years), of delaying the initiation of levodopa therapy (28). Results of a recent study known as Earlier vs Later L-DOPA (ELLDOPA), however, challenge this traditional approach (29).

The ELLDOPA study was a double-blind, placebo-controlled trial designed to assess the effect of levodopa on disease progression in 361 patients with early PD (29). Patients were randomized to receive low-dose high-dose levodopa, or placebo for nine months followed by a 2-week "washout" period (where all patients were taken off their medications). The results showed a greater increase in the severity of parkinsonism in the placebo group compared to the low-dose and high-dose levodopa. However, as high as 25% of the high-dose levodopa group developed fluctuations and/or dyskinesias after only nine months. These clinical results indicated that treatment of patients with levodopa early in the course of disease showed a dose-dependent relief of their symptoms and suggested that delaying initiation of treatment deserved reappraisal. Owing to the short duration (two weeks) of the levodopa washout, it remained unclear whether the early use of levodopa slowed disease progression.

How different is Stalevo from Sinemet?

Sinemet is actually a combination of levodopa and carbidopa. Levodopa is the active ingredient that enters the brain and is converted to dopamine once it arrives at its destination. When levodopa was marketed alone (without the carbidopa), a lot of patients had significant nausea and vomiting. This is because the levodopa was not absorbed in the gut and was converted to dopamine. In the gut, dopamine cannot be absorbed and therefore it cannot enter the brain beyond its "iron curtain" (called the blood-brain barrier) (it can only enter if it is in levodopa form). Unfortunately, when outside the brain, dopamine is an irritant. It causes nausea and vomiting. This is because one area of the brain (called area postrema) is exposed and stimulated, as it is not situated behind the brain's iron curtain. Carbidopa blocks the enzyme that coverts levodopa to dopamine in the gut so that more of it gets absorbed and less of it stays in the gut as dopamine. Since carbidopa has been automatically incorporated with levodopa, there has been less nausea experienced by patients. Sinemet is in fact derived from the Latin words *sin* (meaning "without") and *emet* (meaning "to vomit"). Sinemet therefore means "without vomiting." Of course, this is not always the case, and some patients actually need extra doses of carbidopa than the one that is built in the Sinemet tablet.

It gets even better. Stalevo combines three ingredients: levodopa, carbidopa, plus entacapone. Entacapone blocks another enzyme that breaks down levodopa in the gut. The net result is more levodopa getting absorbed and entering the brain. It is therefore a good drug for those with wearing-off as it prolongs the life of levodopa (30). A double-blind clinical trial known as STalevo Reduction in Dyskinesia Evaluation (STRIDE)-PD to determine if Stalevo is effective in delaying the start of dyskinesias is ongoing, with a goal of enrolling approximately 700 PWPs requiring levodopa therapy.

Why are there different forms of carbidopa/levodopa? Are they really different from each other?

Carbidopa/levodopa is now available in four forms: immediate-release, orally disintegrating, sustained-release tablets, and as an intestinal gel (marketed as Duodopa in Europe). Ideally, levodopa is best taken at least 30 minutes before or 1 to 2 hours after meals to decrease the competition with amino acids for absorption across the small intestine. Medication can be taken with a small nonprotein snack if amino acid competition is a concern and nausea is a problem.

Carbidopa/levodopa in immediate-release form is available in 10/100, 25/100, or 25/250 mg strengths. Dosing is typically initiated at one 25/100 mg tablet three times daily and increased by one pill as necessary until a clinical response is achieved. The recommended maximum doses are 200 mg carbidopa and 2000 mg levodopa per day. Occasionally, the immediate-release form is used to make a liquid preparation for PWPs with significant motor fluctuations by mixing 10 tablets with half teaspoon of ascorbic acid crystals and 1000 mL distilled water. This preparation allows small frequent dosing with the goal of relieving wearing-off symptoms without causing or worsening peak-dose dyskinesias.

Parcopa is an immediate-release, orally disintegrating form of carbidopa/levodopa available in the same dose combinations as the standard tablets. It dissolves underneath the tongue without requiring water. But unlike the orally disintegrating selegiline, it still needs to go through the gut and to get absorbed. Therefore, its onset of action is not much faster than the immediate-release carbidopa/levodopa. Parcopa contains phenylalanine, 3.4 mg in the 10/100 mg and 25/100 mg strengths, and 8.4 mg in the 25/250 mg tablets.

Sustained-release carbidopa/levodopa is available in 25/100 and 50/200 mg strengths. The time it takes to reach peak efficacy is slower than the immediate-release, taking about 2 to 3 hours. Thus, most patients who have been exposed to the immediate-release form do not like the controlled-release form because they do not feel the "kick start" that they usually do when they take the immediate-release formulation. The initial recommended dose is 50/200 mg twice daily, at least 6 hours apart. The dose can be increased every few days up to a theoretical maximum of eight per day, with 4 to 8 hours intervals between administrations. Dose requirements of the controlled-release preparation are usually 10% to 25% higher than regular release levodopa owing to its decreased bioavailability. Absorption is altered by both the stomach acidity and the time it takes for the stomach to empty its contents and pass it on to the small intestines, which may be slower in elderly subjects or in the presence of food. Taking Sinemet CR with protein will also decrease absorption due to competition with amino acids for absorption from the small intestine. Sinemet CR should not be crushed or chewed; otherwise, it functions like an immediate-release tablet.

Finally, carbidopa/levodopa can now be continuously infused in the intestine through a stomach tube. This continuous delivery of levodopa in the form of a liquid gel prevents and relieves motor fluctuations. It is only available in Europe at the time of this writing. There are a few centers in the United States that are offering this formulation but only as part of a research clinical trial. The ideal candidate for the carbidopa-levodopa intestinal gel formulation is a PWP experiencing significant motor fluctuations or dyskinesias despite the best efforts to optimize treatment.

Does levodopa slow the progression of PD?

Levodopa has changed the lives of millions of PWPs. Patients now live longer and have more rewarding lives with much less and even slower progressing disability in some cases (when compared to the prelevodopa era). The positive effects of levodopa can be felt for many years; however, levodopa is not a cure. Levodopa does not relieve all symptoms of PD. In addition, not all patients respond to levodopa with consistent results, although most respond very well. Levodopa may also have side effects—and some patients in the PD population seem to be more susceptible to side effects than others—so therapy needs to be tailored to the individual.

As to whether levodopa slows disease progression in PD, the jury is still out. The data are conflicting. We have a large clinical trial that showed that those on the highest dose of levodopa had the best motor function and the slowest decline. The imaging arm of that study, however, revealed that the basal ganglia (the part of the brain that is sick in PD) had significantly less amounts of surviving dopaminergic brain cells. We have been unable to definitively explain this discrepancy between the clinical finding and the imaging results. Most authorities believe, however, that levodopa does not affect disease progression, but this remains a controversial topic. More research may shed light on this controversy (3,31–39).

I am, unfortunately, experiencing significant motor fluctuations. What are my treatment options?

The overall objectives of managing PWPs are to control symptoms, improve the patients' quality of life, and allow the patients to maintain daily function in a manner that is as close as possible to normal without experiencing side effects from treatment. As mentioned in Chapter 3, as PD symptoms worsen, wearing-off or end-of-dose deterioration become common. One therapeutic option for dealing with wearing-off involves the simple adjustment of levodopa by reducing each individual dose but increasing dose frequency (40). Other options include the addition of pharmacological agents such as dopamine agonists or MAO-B inhibitors, or conversion from a standard immediate-release levodopa formulation to a controlled-release formulation (2,41–43). The time it takes for levodopa to take its effect is about 30 to 90 minutes with standard immediate-release formulations compared with 60 to 180 minutes with controlled-release levodopa (1). A 2002 literature review by PD experts concluded that the choice of immediate-release versus controlled-release levodopa for the initiation of treatment had no affect on the rate of motor complications. However, levodopa therapy should be tailored to the individual patient based on the magnitude and duration of response in the individual after a single dose of levodopa/carbidopa, as well as observation of the relationship between "on" and "off" periods in the patient. For example, we have patients who would experience dyskinesias if given more than one-fourth tablet of Sinemet, so it has to be given at this dose every 2 hours.

What about COMT inhibitors? When should they be used?

Catechol-O-methyltransferase (COMT) is an enzyme that breaks down levodopa while it is still in the gut. Thus, blocking this enzyme decreases the breakdown of levodopa, thereby enhancing its half-life (defined as the amount of time it takes for a drug to lose half of its pharmacological activity) by approximately 26% and consequently increasing the amount of the drug available to the brain (1,27,44,45). COMT inhibitors in combination with levodopa improve end-of-dose wearing off, reduce off time, and increase on time (40,44,46,47).

Because of a few reports of deaths from liver toxicity associated with use of the older COMT inhibitor tolcapone, liver function monitoring is required for the first 6 months of therapy for patients receiving tolcapone. Other adverse events associated with COMT inhibitors include diarrhea, nausea, vomiting, dyskinesia, and hepatotoxicity (tolcapone only) (40,44,46,47). So far, there have been no reports of deaths from liver toxicity with the newer COMT inhibitor, entacapone. Therefore, liver monitoring is not required with entacapone.

The COMT inhibitors tolcapone and entacapone are available for clinical use in the treatment of PD patients experiencing motor fluctuations (especially wearing off) as is the combination tablet (Stalevo) containing the COMT inhibitor entacapone, levodopa, and carbidopa.

What is apomorphine? When should I talk to my doctor about considering this option?

Apomorphine is a soluble, nonergot dopamine receptor agonist just like pramipexole, ropinirole, and rotigotine (44,48). It was recently reported that apomorphine injected subcutaneously (meaning, just underneath the skin) in a specially designed syringe provides effective "rescue" treatment for patients with sudden, unexpected, levodopa-induced off periods (44,46–48). The good news is that the medication works as quickly as 5 to 10 minutes. The bad news is that it only lasts for about 1 to 1.5 hours at the most. Thus, it cannot be used as a mainstay treatment, but it should be used as a rescue therapy that will make the patient comfortable while waiting for the main drugs to kick in. This treatment, however, is associated with a relatively high frequency of side effects including nausea, lightheadedness, yawning, and drowsiness (44). Subcutaneous continuous infusion of apomorphine is now approved in Europe.

Are there drugs that can prevent or slow down PD?

There has long been interest as to whether MAO-B inhibitors may have disease modifying or neuroprotective benefits in PD. Disease modifying agents are thought to alter the course or progression of a particular disease. Neuroprotective therapies alternatively provide protection of neurons from neurodegeneration or other injuries. No therapies to date have been definitively proven to be disease modifying or neuroprotective in PWPs.

At the American Neurological Association meeting in December 2008, results were finally released from the long-awaited Attenuation of Disease Progression with Azilect Given Once daily (ADAGIO) study. The study was a randomized double-blind placebo-controlled trial and had 1176 early PWPs making it even larger than the DATATOP study. The ADAGIO study utilized a novel design called a delayed-start. The results revealed that the 1 mg dose of rasagiline may have had a disease modifying benefit. Specifically, the group randomized to the delayed start of rasagiline therapy failed to "catch up" to those randomized to the immediate start with 1 mg per day of rasagiline. Interestingly, unexpectedly and also without clear explanation, those who received the higher 2 mg rasagiline dose immediately did not do as well as those who received the lower 1 mg dose. The results were also recently presented at the twelfth Congress of the European Federation of Neurological Societies, in Madrid, Spain.

Some of the controversy in interpretation has been centered around the study endpoints, which were based on a common PD scale called the Unified Parkinson's Disease Rating Scale (UPDRS), which has several limitations. The impact of change from baseline of only 1.7 units (combined score with all UPDRS subscores), and the mystery as to why the 2 mg dose did not do as well as the 1 mg dose, has drawn criticism from some experts in the scientific community. The novel study design has also been criticized as potentially falling short of proving the high bar of disease modification or neuroprotection. Finally, it is possible that certain subtypes of PD may have fueled the statistical benefit. We are not able at this time to tease these out (eg, genetic, tremor predominant, etc.) The study ultimately revealed the 1 mg dose to be safe and well tolerated, and because of the novel delayed-start design it can be argued that rasagiline has a possible disease modifying effect.

Almost the identical "delayed-start" clinical trial design was performed this time testing whether the immediate use of pramipexole was advantageous over delayed initiations of the medication. We await the results of this study.

Several other agents are being studied in large scale to determine if they may potentially slow disease progression. These include the natural supplements CoQ10 and creatine, and the antihypertensive isradipine.

What is the best drug for depression?

There is, unfortunately, a paucity of data concerning the use of specific antidepressants in treating depression in PD. While the basis for most treatment has been extrapolated from studies on depression in the non-PD population, a few current PD-specific researches provide some guidance on the treatment of depression in PD. First, studies indicate that PWPs are as responsive to antidepressant treatments as other older adults with depression are. Although one study suggests that amitriptyline (a type of TCA) may be superior to SSRIs, the majority of studies suggest that SSRIs and TCAs are both reasonable options.

The side effect profiles of these medications may be useful in helping the clinician select a particular treatment (Table 5.2). While SSRIs are generally better tolerated than TCAs, there are certain situations in which TCAs may be preferred. For example, TCAs (such as amitriptyline, imipramine, and doxepin) may be beneficial in patients with insomnia, bladder hyperactivity, and drooling because of their anticholinergic effects. In contrast, these anticholinergic properties may worsen cognitive impairment, hallucinations, hypotension, or excessive daytime somnolence. Depressed patients with comorbid anxiety may also respond better to SSRIs, since these drugs are approved for use in both conditions.

Other medications that have been found efficacious in the treatment of depression in PD include nefazodone, mirtazapine, and even dopamine agonists. Both nefazodone and mirtazapine may be useful in the patient who is also suffering from insomnia. Studies have also suggested that mirtazapine may improve tremor and dyskinesias in some patients (49). Pramipexole has been shown to improve depression in PWPs and patients without PD. A recent clinical trial demonstrated that pramipexole had a significantly higher response rate than sertraline (one of the most popular SSRIs) in treating depression in PD (50). Studies have also found ropinirole to improve depression in PWPs.

Table 5.2 Side Effects of Antidepressants Used in Parkinson's Disease

Drug	Dose (mg/d)	Sedation	Drop in blood pressure	Antimuscarinic effects (eg, dry mouth, blurred vision, heart rhythm effects, etc.)	Sexual dysfunction	Weight gain
Fluoxetine	10–80	Negligible	Negligible	Negligible	Considerable	Mild
Fluvoxamine	50–300	Negligible	Negligible	Negligible	Moderate	Moderate
Paroxetine	20–50	Mild	Negligible	Mild	Severe	Moderate
Sertraline	25–100	Negligible	Negligible	Negligible	Moderate	Mild
Citalopram	10–60	Mild	Negligible	Mild	Moderate	Mild
Escitalopram	10–20	Mild	Negligible	Mild	Moderate	Mild
Amitriptyline	25–200	Considerable	Moderate	Considerable	Mild	Considerable
Doxepine	75–150	Moderate	Moderate	Considerable	Mild	Moderate
Imipramine	50–200	Moderate	Considerable	Moderate	Mild	Moderate
Desipramine	100–300	Mild	Mild	Mild	Negligible	Mild
Nortriptyline	50–150	Mild	Mild	Mild	Negligible	Mild
Buproprion	150–450	Negligible	Negligible	Mild	Negligible	Negligible
Mirtazepine	15–45	Moderate	Moderate	Mild	Moderate	Considerable
Nefazodone	300–600	Moderate	Moderate	Negligible	Mild	Negligible
Venlafaxine	75–375	Mild	Negligible	Mild	Considerable	Mild

Source: From Ref. 51.

As a caution, certain medications should be avoided in the PWP. Amoxapine and lithium both have the potential to cause or worsen parkinsonism, and nonselective MAOIs can lead to a hypertensive crisis in PWPs on levodopa.

Are there drugs available to help improve concentration and memory in PD?

First, before starting any treatment to enhance cognition, a full work-up for treatable conditions of cognitive impairment should be performed. The knee-jerk reaction of attributing everything to PD should be resisted. Diagnostic work-up may include a brain imaging study, a complete metabolic panel, thyroid studies, vitamin B12 level, and serological studies for slow growing infections (such as syphilis). A careful review of the patient's medications, including nonprescription medications, frequently reveals contributors to the patient's cognitive decline (such as antihistamines and anticholinergic agents). A precipitous decline in cognition may be an indicator of an acute infection (eg, urinary tract infection or pneumonia) or social stressor such as moving (51).

Cholinesterase inhibitors (such as rivastigmine, donepezil, and galantamine) and memantine have been shown to slow the progression and improve the cognitive and behavioral profile of AD patients. Cholinesterase inhibitors are believed to work by increasing brain levels of acetylcholine, which is an important neurotransmitter for memory that is also affected by PD. One large clinical trial of rivastigmine in PD with dementia has demonstrated improvements in cognition, activities of daily living, and neuropsychiatric complications (52). Smaller trials and experience in AD suggest that donepezil and galantamine may also be reasonable options. Tacrine, the oldest of all cholinesterase inhibitors, is rarely used due to its risk of hepatotoxicity and its frequent dosing. For all the cholinesterase inhibitors, the most common side effects are gastrointestinal distress (nausea, diarrhea, vomiting), fatigue, nightmares, insomnia, and muscle cramps. The rates of these complications may be higher in PWPs but are often mild. Gastrointestinal symptoms typically resolve with time and may be minimized by taking the medication with food, especially fatty food. Increased tremor may also be seen but this is typically mild and transient.

There have been no clinical trials of memantine in the treatment of dementia in PD. One small study has shown it to be safe in PD and possibly improve parkinsonian symptoms (53). As PD dementia frequently cooccurs with AD pathology it may be a reasonable choice for patients with moderate to severe dementia. Side effects of memantine include headache, constipation, and confusion.

What medications can be used to treat psychosis in PD?

Just like the management of cognitive decline, prior to starting any treatment, one has to search for urinary tract infections, pneumonia, metabolic derangements, sleep disturbances, brain insults (such as strokes), and social stressors, such as changes in the environment, as possible explanations for hallucinations or delusions. Medications that can alter brain mechanics because of their ability to penetrate the brain's "iron curtain" (termed the "blood brain barrier") that is designed to keep away unwanted substances, such as narcotics, hypnotics, antidepressants, and anxiolytics are also common culprits. If psychotic symptoms persist despite the withdrawal of other psychotropic medications, anti-PD medications may be gradually reduced or, if necessary, discontinued. As mentioned in Chapter 4, most authorities recommend "peeling off" these medications in the following order: anticholinergic agents, amantadine, MAOIs, dopamine agonists, COMT inhibitors, and finally, levodopa (53). Regular or short-acting formulations of levodopa are preferred in patients prone to hallucinations over sustained-release formulations because their pharmacokinetics are more predictable and there is less potential for cumulative side effects. If psychosis improves, the patient is then maintained on the lowest possible dose of anti-PD medications. However, if the withdrawal of anti-PD drugs significantly worsens other PD symptoms or does not control psychosis one must consider the addition of antipsychotic agents.

The choice of an antipsychotic agent is largely based on its ease of use and side effect profile, as most antipsychotics have comparable efficacy in improving psychosis. Atypical antipsychotics (or newer generation antipsychotics) are generally preferred given the significant risk of motor complications and anticholinergic side effects with older, conventional antipsychotics (54–60). The use of an appropriate atypical antipsychotic agent may allow the clinician to control psychosis with fewer motor side effects and, in some cases, without the need for significantly cutting back on anti-PD medications. Clinicians should be aware that the FDA issued a "black box" warning for the use of these agents in the treatment of psychosis associated with dementia due to increased cardiac mortality. However, the majority of clinicians treating these patients continue to use these medications because these medications are efficacious, the absolute risk of increased mortality is low, and the risk appears to be present in the older antipsychotics as well (61,62).

The main difference in the antipsychotics lies in their propensity to worsen motor functioning in this frail and already vulnerable population. Quetiapine has been studied in PWPs and appears to have less potential for worsening motor function than risperidone, aripiprazole, olanzapine, and ziprasidone. While double-blinded trials of quetiapine have been disappointing, it remains the first-line agent used for drug-induced psychosis in Parkinson's due to its tolerability and good track record in several open-label trials (54–60,63).

The use of clozapine is generally limited to patients who have failed other agents, despite its superior efficacy over all other antipsychotic drugs, because of its very uncommon risk of agranulocytosis (meaning, sudden drop in white blood cell count—our body's first defense against ordinary infections). The chances of this complication developing are less than 1%. Nonetheless, in the United States, for the first 6 months, each patient on clozapine must undergo a weekly white blood cell count and can receive only one week's supply of the drug at a time. After 6 months, the process becomes biweekly.

It remains unclear how long antipsychotic medications should be continued once they are initiated. There are some data that show persistence of hallucinations in PWPs with drug-induced psychosis after its initial occurrence. At the University of Florida, we prospectively followed our own PWPs on successful long-term treatment with quetiapine or clozapine to see if they could be successfully weaned off their antipsychotic drugs (60). The study was aborted after enrollment of only six patients due to an unacceptably high rate of psychosis recurrence (five patients, 83%).

Other treatment options include acetylcholinesterase inhibitors, odansetron (a rather expensive antinausea medication used mainly for patients undergoing chemotherapy), and ECT. Several open-label studies have found that cholinesterase inhibitors may improve hallucinations and psychosis in PD subjects (64). Similarly, an open-label trial with 16 PWPs showed marked improvements in the areas of visual hallucinations, confusion, and functional impairment with no adverse effects on motor function (65). This result has yet to be reproduced by other investigators. ECT should be reserved for patients who are unresponsive to, or intolerant of, other treatments, especially if the psychosis is associated with severe depression. In general, ECT's effects are short-lived, and repeated treatments and/or the help of other medications are required to maintain benefits.

How are impulse control and compulsive disorders treated?

As mentioned in Chapter 4, examples of impulse control disorders seen in PD include pathological gambling, hypersexuality, compulsive shopping, excessive spending, and binge eating. Examples of compulsive behaviors include compulsive dopaminergic medication use and punding—a stereotyped motor behavior in which there is an intense fascination with repetitive handling and examining of mechanical objects, such as taking apart and reassembling appliances or sorting common objects, like pebbles and jewelry.

The management of these behaviors typically includes decreasing or discontinuing dopamine agonist therapy (for impulse control disorders), lowering the overall dosage of PD medications, or the addition of an atypical antipsychotic drug (for compulsive behavior). However, there have been a few reports of worsening of punding with quetiapine use (66). Occasionally, clomipramine and other SSRIs may alleviate punding. Referrals for specific treatments (eg, gambling treatment) or the use of behavioral interventions may also be helpful and should not be overlooked.

My husband has difficulty staying asleep at night, yet sleeps most of the day. Is there a good medication for his condition?

PWPs are affected by their disease 24 hours of the day, although most clinicians often focus mainly on the waking hours. Appropriate dosages of dopaminergic medication at bedtime may help relieve stiffness and difficulty turning in bed at night, pain, early morning dystonia, and wearing-off symptoms, which can result in improved sleep. Controlled-release preparations are superior to immediate-release levodopa for decreasing sleep disturbances (67). However, excessive dopaminergic medication at night can lead to dyskinesias, hallucinations, and confusion, which can also interfere with normal sleep. Similarly, adequate treatment of depression and anxiety may improve sleep.

If the cause of sleep disturbance is not found, clinicians may consider other drug treatments. Melatonin (50 mg) has been found to benefit PWPs and has fewer side effects than most other pharmacological sleep preparations (68). The use of hypnotics (including over the counter preparations) should be approached cautiously, as these formulations can cause confusion and daytime cognitive problems. Daily use of these medications may also disrupt sleep and lead to withdrawal symptoms or rebound insomnia.

How are restless legs and other sleep disorders associated with PD treated?

For most patients with restless legs syndrome, using low-dose dopamine agonists 30 to 60 minutes before bedtime are the most effective treatments.

Table 5.3 Pharmacological Treatment of Sleep Disorders in Parkinson's Disease

Sleep disturbance	Pharmacological treatments that you can discuss with your doctor
Nocturnal PD symptoms (dystonia, rigidity at night)	Nocturnal dose of continuous release carbidopa/levodopa (for all other symptoms)
Restless legs syndrome	Dopamine agonist at bedtime
	May consider carbidopa/levodopa at bedtime
	Opiates, gabapentin, clonazepam
Rapid eye movement sleep behavior disorder	Clonazepam start 0.5 mg at bedtime may increase to 1–2 mg)
	May consider other benzodiazepines, melatonin
Excessive daytime sleepiness	(Do not take these medications after dinner)
	Methylphenidate start 5 mg 4 times per day
	Amantadine 100 mg twice per day
	Modafenil 50–100 mg once daily
Obstructive sleep apnea	Positive pressure airway ventilation (CPAP/BiPAP)
Depression	Antidepressants, particularly mirtazapine, nefazodone, and tricyclic antidepressants
Nocturia (frequent urination at night)	Tricyclic antidepressants
Hallucinations	Quetiapine start 25–50 mg at bedtime
Primary insomnia	Melatonin 50 mg at bedtime

Alternative treatments include controlled-release levodopa, clonazepam, neurontin, and opiates.

RBD in PD—characterized by vigorous (and sometimes injurious) behavior in REM sleep that usually represents enactment of vivid, action-filled, and/or violent dreams—are almost always relieved with low-dose clonazepam (starting with 0.5–1 mg at bedtime).

As described in Chapter 4, short naps (15–30 minutes) may be helpful in patients with excessive daytime sleepiness, but they should not be taken too late in the day as they may interfere with sleep at night. Stimulant medications such as modafinil, methylphenidate, caffeine, or dextroamphetamine may be also helpful. These medications should not be given later in the day, as they may exacerbate or cause sleep disturbances. Table 5.3 summarizes the sleep disorders and their treatment.

What pharmacological treatments are available for the management of autonomic problems in PD?

Table 5.4 summarizes the currently used drug therapies to alleviate some of the *autonomic problems* seen in PD.

Table 5.4 Treatments of Autonomic Dysfunction in Parkinson's Disease

Symptom	Pharmacological treatments that you can discuss with your doctor
Orthostatic hypotension	Fludrocortisone 0.1 mg once daily
	Midodrine 5–10 mg three times per day; last dose should not be after 6 pm to avoid supine hypertension
	Ephedrine 25–50 mg q4–6 hours
	Phenylpropanolamine start 25 mg twice per day or ergotamine/caffeine tablets; do not take after dinner to avoid insomnia and supine hypertension
	May consider physostigmine, erythropoietin, or octreotide
Constipation	Stool softeners (eg, docusate sodium 50–200 mg daily)
	Osmotic laxatives (lactulose, milk of magnesia)
	Stimulant laxative (bisacodyl) 10–15 mg daily; 10 mg per rectum daily; or 30 ml fleet enema
Excessive drooling	Trihexyphenidyl 2.0–5.0 mg three times per day
	Benztropine 0.5–1.0 mg three times per day
	Glycopyrrolate 1.0–2.0 mg three to four times per day
	Botulinum toxin type A or B: injection over parotid and salivary gland
Erectile dysfunction	Sildenafil 50–100 mg 1 hour prior to intercourse; watch for orthostatic hypotension
	Vardenafil 5–20 mg 1 hour prior to intercourse
	Tadalafil 5–20 mg 1 hour prior to intercourse
	Yohimbine 5–10 mg tid
	Papaverine 1–4 ml of 30mg/ml solution intracavernous injection
Urinary frequency (hyperactive bladder)	Tolterodine 2 mg bid
	Oxybutynin 5 mg tid; patch every 3 days
	Propantheline 15–30 mg four times per day
	Hyoscyamine 0.15–0.3 mg at bedtime, up to four times per day
	Imipramine 10–25 mg at bedtime
	Trospium chloride 20 mg at bedtime
Urinary retention (hypoactive bladder)	Terazosin start 1 mg at bedtime
	Doxazosin 1–4 mg once daily
	Prazosin 1 mg bid or tid; may increase slowly up to 20 mg/day
	Tamsulosin 0.4–0.8 mg once daily
	Bethanechol chloride 10–50 mg three to four times per day; 2.5–5 mg s.c. three to four times per day
Drenching sweats/ diaphoresis	Sinemet CR at bedtime or addition of COMT inhibitor
	Propranolol (start 40 mg twice per day for short-acting 80 mg daily long acting
	Clonidine(start with 0.1 mg/day

Are there medications that we should avoid in PD?

Definitely, clinicians, patients, and caregivers should be aware of potential drug interactions or medications that may worsen PD symptoms. Some drugs should not be used at all, while others must be used cautiously. Table 5.5 lists medications that block dopamine, thereby potentially increasing PD symptoms. In addition, there are several medications that should not be used with MAO-B inhibitors due to an increased risk of high blood pressure, increased heart rate, seizures, fever, or confusion (Tables 5.6 and 5.7).

My doctor is asking me if I would like to participate in a drug study. He calls it a clinical trial and he tells me there is a 50% chance of receiving a sugar pill. Why should I participate?

If you are able and your time allows it, participating in a clinical trial is perhaps one of the best things you can do for yourself and for others. A

Table 5.5 Medications That Should Be Avoided Because They Block or Decrease Dopamine and Can Worsen Parkinson's Symptoms

Antipsychotic medications	Haloperidol (Haldol)
	Loxapine (Loxitane)
	Molindone (Moban)
	Thiothixene (Navane)
	Chlorpromazine (Thorazine)
	Flufenazine (Prolixin)
	Perphenazine (Trilafon)
	Trifluoperazine (Stelazine)
	Thioridazine (Mellaril)
	Risperidone (Risperdal)
	Ziprasidone (Geodon)
	Olanzapine (Zyprexa)
	Aripiprazole (Abilify)
Antidepressants	Amoxapine (Ascendin)
	Perphenazine/amitriptyline (Triavil)
Antiemetics	Prochlorperazine (Compazine)
	Metoclopramide (Reglan)
	Thiethylperazide (Torecan)
	Promethazine (Phenergan)
	Droperidol (Inapsine)
Antihypertensives	Reserpine (Serpasil)
	Rauwolfia serpentina (Raudixin)
	Alpha-methyldopa (Aldomet)

Source: From Ref. 69.

Table 5.6 Medications That Should Not Be Taken in Combination With Levodopa

Antidepressants	Phenelzine (Nardil)
	Tranylcypromine (Parnate)
Iron supplements	May decrease the absorption of levodopa so should be taken at least 2 hours before or after carbidopa/levodopa

Source: From Ref. 69.

clinical trial is a study that involves humans and investigates whether a drug, agent, intervention, or procedure is beneficial for a specific population (in this case, the PD population). When the drug is still tested on rats and monkeys, it is in the preclinical stage. Hundreds of agents are tested in animals, and only a few really make it to the human stage.

Once it reaches the human level, clinical trials generally proceed in three phases: I, II, and III, before it is approved for general consumption by the FDA. Phase I involves testing the drug among healthy, young volunteers (such as college students who would like to make some money for their spring break). The main purpose of phase I is to test whether the medication is well tolerated and generally safe. Phase II involves testing the drug in a small (less than 100) number of patients afflicted with the disease. The main purposes of phase II are to test if the drug is safe in the population being studied and to get an idea of the best dose to be tested in phase III. Thus, a typical design for a phase II trial is a "dose ranging design." Phase III is the last step before the FDA considers the drug for marketing. Phase III involves testing of the drug in large numbers of patients afflicted with the disease (typically 200 to 300 patients). The main purposes of a phase III study are to determine efficacy and to ensure continued safety. Usually, the FDA will require at least two positive phase III studies before it deliberates on the merits of the drug. To be sure that

Table 5.7 Medications That Should Not be Used, or Used Very Cautiously, With MAO-B Inhibitors Selegiline (Eldepryl, Zelapar) and Rasagiline (Azilect)

The narcotic meperidine (Demerol) should not be used at all. Patients should be taught to notify health care providers before surgery or colonoscopy is scheduled. The antidepressant mirtazipine (Remeron) and St Johns wort should be avoided, if possible.
Cough medicines containing dextromethorphan should be avoided, if possible.
Cold, allergy, and sinus medications containing pseudophedrine (Sudafed) and ephedrine should be avoided, if possible.

Source: From Ref. 69.

the drug really works, there should be a difference in the effect on patients who receive the real drug versus those who receive a sugar pill (thus it is called placebo-controlled); everyone should have an equal chance of receiving the real drug or placebo (that is why it is *randomized*); and not one center can enroll all 300 hundred patients (so it is often a multicenter trial). Everyone helps out, the clinicians, the industry sponsor, the government, and the patients. Once the drug is approved and available for patients, any postmarketing studies are labeled phase IV clinical trials.

So now we hope you realize that in order for a single drug to make it to the market, it has to go through many hurdles, and hundreds of patients (and healthy volunteers) need to participate. Once a drug reaches the human or clinical trial phase, it takes anywhere from 8 to 10 years before it eventually becomes available in the drug stores. And only 1 out of 10 medications that reach phase I will eventually cross the finish line, ie, have two successful phase III trials, and get approved by the FDA. The progress of medicine may seem slow to the person suffering from the illness, but this process has been tried and tested. We can speed up a few steps, but the general process has to be kept in place to make sure that a drug is truly efficacious and safe for all. Sometimes, despite the scientific rigor applied in conducting the trials, things fall through the cracks…drugs still get pulled out of the market because of unforeseen side effects…remember pergolide?

We always tell our patients, "the reason why you have more options now than your father had a decade ago is because 10 years ago, your father's friend volunteered to participate in a clinical trial. And the reason why your son will have even more hope tomorrow is because, today, you participated in a clinical trial."

REFERENCES

1. Tetrud J. Treatment challenges in early stage Parkinson's disease. *Neurol Clin*. 2004;22(3 suppl):S19–S33.
2. Guttman M, Kish SJ, Furukawa Y. Current concepts in the diagnosis and management of Parkinson's disease. *CMAJ*. 2003;168:292–301.
3. Olanow CW. The scientific basis for the current treatment of Parkinson's disease. *Annu Rev Med*. 2004;55:41–60.
4. Rascol O. Rasagiline in the pharmacotherapy of Parkinson's disease-a review. *Expert Opin Pharmacother*. 2005;6:2061–2075.
5. Olanow CW, Watts RL, Koller WC. An algorithm (decision tree) for the management of Parkinson's disease: treatment guidelines. *Neurology*. 2001;56(suppl 5):S1–S88.

6. Rascol O, Brooks DJ, Korczyn AD, De Deyn PP, Clarke CE, Lang AE. A five-year study of the incidence of dyskinesia in patients with early Parkinson's disease who were treated with ropinirole or levodopa. *N Engl J Med.* 2000;342:1484–1491.

7. Schapira AH, Obeso J. Timing of treatment initiation in Parkinson's disease: a need for reappraisal? *Ann Neurology.* 2006;59:559–562.

8. Crosby N, Deane KHO, Clarke CE. Amantadine in Parkinson's disease [review]. *The Cochrane Database of Systematic Reviews.* 2003; 1: Art. No.CD003468.

9. Lang AE, Lees A. Amantadine and other antiglutamate agents. *Mov Disord.* 2002;17:S13–S22.

10. Pahwa R, Factor SA, Lyons KE, et al. Practice parameter: treatment of Parkinson disease with motor fluctuations and dyskinesia (an evidence-based review): report of the Quality Standards Subcommittee of the American Academy of Neurology. *Neurology.* 2006;66:983–995.

11. Katzenschlager R, Sampaio C, Costa J, Lee A. Anticholinergics for symptomatic management of Parkinson's disease [review]. *Cochrane Database Syst Rev.* 2005;4:1–18.

12. Parkinson Study Group. DATATOP: a multicenter controlled clinical trial in early Parkinson's disease. *Arch Neurol.* 1989;46:1052–1060.

13. Shoulson I. Deprenyl and tocopherol antioxidative therapy of parkinsonism (DATATOP). Parkinson Study Group. *Acta Neurol Scand Suppl.* 1989;126:171–175.

14. Macleod AD, Counsell CE, Stowe R. Monoamine oxidase B inhibitors for early Parkinson's disease [review]. *The Cochrane Database of Systematic Reviews.* 2005;3: Art. No.CD004898.

15. LeWitt PA. Clinical trials of neuroprotection for Parkinson's disease. *Neurology.* 2004;63:S23–S31.

16. Shoulson I, Oakes D, Fahn S, et al. Impact of sustained deprenyl (selegiline) in levodopa-treated Parkinson's disease: a randomized placebo-controlled extension of the deprenyl and tocopherol antioxidative therapy of parkinsonism trial. *Ann Neurol.* 2002;51:604–612.

17. Stern MB, Marek KL, Friedman J, et al. Double-blind, randomized, controlled trial of rasagiline as monotherapy in early Parkinson's disease patients. *Mov Disord.* 2004;19:916–923.

18. Parkinson Study Group. A controlled trial of rasagiline in early Parkinson disease: the TEMPO Study. *Arch Neurol.* 2002;59:1937–1943.

19. Parkinson Study Group. A controlled, randomized, delayed-start study of rasagiline in early Parkinson disease. *Arch Neurol.* 2004;61:561–566.

20. Parkinson Study Group. A randomized placebo-controlled trial of rasagiline in levodopa-treated patients with Parkinson disease and motor fluctuations: the PRESTO study. *Arch Neurol.* 2005;62:241–248.

21. Rascol O, Brooks DJ, Melamed E, et al.; for the LARGO Study Group. Rasagiline as an adjunct to levodopa in patients with Parkinson's disease and

motor fluctuations (LARGO, lasting effect in adjunct therapy with rasagiline given once daily, study): a randomised, double-blind, parallel-group trial. *Lancet.* 2005;365:947–954.

22. Richard IH, Kurlan R, Tanner C, et al. Serotonin syndrome and the combined use of deprenyl and an antidepressant in Parkinson's disease. *Neurology.* 1997;48:1070–1077.

23. Panisset M, Schwid S, Ondo W, Fitzer-Attas C, Chen JJ. Safety of concomitant therapy with rasagiline and antidepressants in Parkinson's disease [abstract in *Mov Disord.* 2007;223(suppl 16):S104–S105]. Presented at the Annual Meeting of the Movement Disorder Society, 2007.

24. Seager H. Drug-delivery products and the Zydis fast-dissolving dosage form. *J Pharm Pharmacol.* 1998;50:375–382.

25. Clarke A, Brewer F, Johnson ES, et al. A new formulation of selegiline: improved bioavailability and selectivity for MAO-B inhibition. *J Neural Transm.* 2003;110:1241–1255.

26. Parkinson Study Group. Pramipexole vs levodopa as initial treatment for Parkinson disease: a randomized controlled trial. *JAMA.* 2000;284:1931–1938.

27. Rascol O, Payoux P, Ory F, Ferriera JJ, Brefel-Courbon C, Montastruc J-L. Limitations of current Parkinson's disease therapy. *Ann Neurol.* 2003;53:S3–S15.

28. Schapira AH, Olanow CW. Rationale for the use of dopamine agonists as neuroprotective agents in Parkinson's disease. *Ann Neurol.* 2003;53(suppl 3):S149–S157.

29. Parkinson Study Group. Levodopa and the progression of Parkinson's disease. *N Engl J Med.* 2004;351:2498–2508.

30. Hauser RA. Levodopa/carbidopa/entacapone (Stalevo). *Neurology.* 2004;62(suppl 1):S64–S71.

31. Clarke, CE. Neuroprotection and pharmacotherapy for motor symptoms in Parkinson's disease. *Lancet Neurol.* 2004;3(8):466–474.

32. Castro AF, Valldeoriola, et al. Optimization of use of levodopa in Parkinson's disease: role of levodopa-carbidopa-entacapone combination [in Portugese]. *Neurologia.* 2005.

33. Fahn S. Does levodopa slow or hasten the rate of progression of Parkinson's disease? *J Neurol.* 2005;252(suppl 4):IV37–IV42.

34. Fahn S. A new look at levodopa based on the ELLDOPA study. *J Neural Transm Suppl.* 2006;(70):419–426.

35. Fahn, S. Levodopa in the treatment of Parkinson's disease. *J Neural Transm Suppl.* 2006;(71):1–15.

36. Suchowersky O, Gronseth G, et al. Practice parameter: neuroprotective strategies and alternative therapies for Parkinson disease (an evidence-based review). Report of the Quality Standards Subcommittee of the American Academy of Neurology. *Neurology.* 2006;

37. Chan PL, Nutt JG, et al. Levodopa slows progression of Parkinson's disease: external validation by clinical trial simulation. *Pharm Res.* 2007;24(4):791–802.

38. Schapira AH. Future directions in the treatment of Parkinson's disease. *Mov Disord.* 2007;22(suppl 17):S385–S391.

39. LeWitt PA, Taylor DC. Protection against Parkinson's disease progression: clinical experience. *Neurotherapeutics.* 2008;5(2):210–225.

40. Bhidayasiri R, Truong DD. Motor complications in Parkinson disease: clinical manifestations and management. *J Neurol Sci.* 2008;266:204–215.

41. Jankovic J. An update on the treatment of Parkinson's disease. *Mt Sinai J Med.* 2006;73:682–689.

42. Grosset DG, Grosset KA, Okun MS, Fernandez HH. *Clinician's Desk Reference: Parkinson's Disease.* London: Manson; 2009.

43. Fernandez HH, Rodriguez RL, Skidmore FM, Okun MS. *A Practical Approach to Any Movement Disorder: Diagnosis, Medical and Surgical Management.* New York, NY: Demos; 2007.

44. Jankovic J, Stacy M. Medical management of levodopa-associated motor complications in patients with Parkinson's disease. *CNS Drugs.* 2007;21:677–692.

45. Rao SS, Hofmann LA, Shakil A. Parkinson's disease: diagnosis and treatment. *Am Fam Physician.* 2006;74:2046–2054.

46. Pahwa R. Understanding Parkinson's disease: an update on current diagnostic and treatment strategies. *J Am Med Dir Assoc.* 2006;7:1–20.

47. Pahwa R, Factor SA, Lyons KE, et al. Practice parameter: treatment of Parkinson disease with motor fluctuations and dyskinesia (an evidence-based review): report of the Quality Standards Subcommittee of the American Academy of Neurology. *Neurology.* 2006;66:983–995.

48. Radad K, Gille G, Rausch WD. Short review on dopamine agonists: insight into clinical and research studies relevant to Parkinson's disease. *Pharmacol Reports.* 2005;57:701–712.

49. Pact V, Giduz T. Mirtazapine treats resting tremor, essential tremor, and levodopa-induced dyskinesias. *Neurology.* 1999;53(5):1154.

50. Barone P, Scarzella L, Marconi R, et al. Pramipexole versus sertraline in the treatment of depression in Parkinson's disease: a national multicenter parallel-group randomized study. *J Neurol.* 2006;253(5):601–607.

51. Kluger BM, Fernandez HH. Management of non-motor manifestations of Parkinson's disease. In: Simuni T, Pahwa R, eds. *Parkinson's Disease.* New York, NY: Oxford University Press; 2009:83–94.

52. Emre M, Aarsland D, Albanese A, et al. Rivastigmine for dementia associated with Parkinson's disease. *N Engl J Med.* 2004;351(24):2509–2518.

53. Merello M, Nouzeilles MI, Cammarota A, et al. Effect of memantine (NMDA antagonist) on Parkinson's disease: a double-blind crossover randomized study. *Clin Neuropharmacol.* 1999;22(5):273–276.

54. Friedman JH, Fernandez HH. Non-motor problems in Parkinson's disease. *Neurolog.* 2000;6(1):18–27.

55. Fernandez HH, Friedman JH, Jacques C, Rosenfeld M. Quetiapine for the treatment of drug-induced psychosis in Parkinson's disease. *Mov Disord.* 1999;14(3):484–487.

56. Fernandez HH, Friedman JH, Lannon MC, Abbott BP. Clozapine replacement by quetiapine for drug-induced psychosis in Parkinson's disease. *Mov Disord.* 2000;3:579–581.

57. Fernandez HH, Trieschmann ME, Burke MA, Friedman JH. Quetiapine use for psychosis in Parkinson disease versus dementia with Lewy bodies. *Journal of Clinical Psychiatry.* 2002;63(6):513–515.

58. Fernandez HH, Trieschmann ME, Friedman JH. The treatment of psychosis in Parkinson's disease: safety considerations. *Drug Safety.* 2003;26 (9):643–659.

59. Fernandez HH, Trieschmann ME, Friedman JH. Aripiprazole for drug induced psychosis in Parkinson's disease: preliminary experience. *Clinical Neuropharmacology.* 2004;27:4–5.

60. Fernandez HH, Trieschmann ME, Okun MS. Rebound psychosis: effect of discontinuation of antipsychotics in Parkinson's disease. *Mov Disord.* 2005;20(1):104–105.

61. Friedman JH. Atypical antipsychotics in the elderly with Parkinson disease and the "black box" warning. *Neurology.* 2006;67(4):564–566.

62. Fernandez HH, Trieschmann ME, Burke MA, Jacques C, Friedman JH. Long-term quetiapine use for drug-induced psychosis among Parkinsonian patients. *Mov Disord.* 2003;18(5):510–514.

63. Wint DP, Okun MS, Fernandez HH. Psychosis in Parkinson's disease. *J Geriatr Psychiatry Neurol.* 2004;17(3):127–136.

64. Hanagasi HA, Emre M. Treatment of behavioural symptoms and dementia in Parkinson's disease. *Fundam Clin Pharmacol.* 2005;19(2):133–146.

65. Zoldan J, Friedberg G, Livneh M, et al. Psychosis in advanced Parkinson's disease: treatment with ondansetron, a 5-HT3 receptor antagonist. *Neurology.* 1995;45(7):1305–1308.

66. Miwa H, Morita S, Nakanshi I, et al. Stereotyped behaviors or punding after quetiapine administration in Parkinson's disease. *Parkinsonism Relat Disord.* 2004;10(3):177–180.

67. Pahwa R, Busenbark, Huber SJ, et al. Clinical experience with controlled-release carbidopa/levodopa in Parkinson's disease. *Neurology.* 1993;43(4):677–681.

68. Dowling GA, Mastick J, Colling E, et al. Melatonin for sleep disturbances in Parkinson's disease. *Sleep Med.* 2005;6(5):459–466.

69. Tuite PJ, Thomas CA, Rukert LF, Fernandez HH. *Parkinson's Disease: A Guide to Patient Care.* New York, NY: Springer; 2009.

I recently was diagnosed with the early stages of Parkinson's disease. I have declined an opportunity to enter a clinical study because I am still trying to work 50 hours a week and felt that the possible complications of the drug might cause me to miss work (which I cannot do at this stage of my life.) I have an extremely stressful job and am finding it difficult to work due to stiffness, concentration problems, aches, and shakiness. The neurologist that I saw said that I could go on meds if I wanted to but that was a decision that I needed to make. Instead of trying the meds that the neurologist offered, I have decided to try a more "natural" approach first. I have seen a physical therapist and received some instructions on exercises that I can do. I am morbidly obese (300 lbs) and have made an appointment with a registered dietician. I have gotten some books on Parkinson's disease so that I can find out more about it and also went to see my general doctor to find about vitamin supplements and CoQ10. She suggested a "regular vitamin" would be good enough and that the CoQ10 was included in most vitamins. When I went to buy the vitamins, I found this not to be true—at least not at the pharmacy I went to. So, I bought a bottle of 200 mg CoQ10 and a bottle of a multivitamin containing vitamin B_6 and B_{12} mcg of B_{12}. Is this a good enough start?

CHAPTER 6

Alternative and Complementary Approaches to Treatment

How often are alternative or complementary medications used in PD? How are they different from conventional drugs?

With the widespread utilization of the Internet, the use of complementary therapies by PWPs has dramatically risen. Even as early as a decade ago, a study showed that 40% of PWPs utilized complementary therapies including vitamins, herbs, massage, and acupuncture (1). Unfortunately, little scientific evidence existed regarding the safety and efficacy of most of these alternative treatments.

Twelve years ago, the out-of-pocket conservative expenditures for complementary medicine in PWPs in the United States reached 27 billion dollars.

The use of herbal remedies and nutritional supplements is governed, in the United States, by the 1994 Dietary Supplement and Health Education Act. This act exempts the companies manufacturing these products from having to provide detailed safety and efficacy information. In Europe, most vitamins, minerals, and supplements are classified and treated as "foods" and medicinal claims are not permitted. Nutrient contents are declared according to the European Union Recommended Daily Allowances (2).

Just because a product is "natural" does not mean that it is always safe. The National Center for Complementary and Alternative Medicine in the United States has been funding studies of common herbal medications to examine drug interactions (3). As an example, Hu and coworkers (4) reported that the use of piper methysticum (more popularly known as "kava") actually increased the off periods in PWPs taking levodopa. In the United Kingdom, the Foundation for Integrated Health has argued for combining complementary and alternative approaches with mainstream medicine.

Instead of taking synthetic dopamine (Sinemet), can I just chew Mucuna pruriens a few times a day?

Mucuna pruriens is the seed powder of a leguminous plant. Leguminous plants belong to the family including peas, beans, clover, alfalfa, and other plants. *Mucuna* was used in ancient Indian medicine as a treatment for PD symptoms. There was a recent article in the *Journal of Neurology Neurosurgery and Psychiatry* that demonstrated that *Mucuna* had a faster effect and higher peak doses when compared to standard Sinemet. There was a similar overall clinical effect to standard Sinemet. Therefore, if one can obtain pharmaceutical grade *Mucuna* (reliable manufacturing process) it can be effective against the symptoms of PD (5–6).

The major challenge is determining the exact amount of *Mucuna* that would be equivalent to a tablet of Sinemet or getting a consistent amount of *Mucuna* with each dose. Just because one takes the same amount of ounces of power, it does not mean that it contains the same amount of the active ingredient. In addition, with so many companies offering *Mucuna* on the Internet, it is hard to tell which ones are "pharmacy-grade" and which ones are not.

Is acupuncture really beneficial in PD? My neighbor swears by it.

Acupuncture started in China and has been practiced for over 3000 years. It strives to balance "yin and yang." However, its biological mechanism of action is yet to be properly defined. Anecdotal patient reports include temporary benefits in tremor and stiffness. However, it is not completely free from side effects. Although rare, complications may include the risk of hepatitis B virus transmission, bacterial endocarditis (infection of the heart valves), spinal infection, osteomyelitis (infection of the bones), compartment syndrome (constriction of vessels, nerves, muscles because of significant swelling in a confined space), cardiac tamponade (a life threatening condition where the heart is unable to pump properly because of too much surrounding blood or fluid thereby constricting the heart), pneumothorax (air pushing the lungs), and spinal cord and root injuries.

Unfortunately, most reported studies of acupuncture are "open label" (meaning, both the patient and the clinician knows that the patient is getting the real thing). This is somewhat understandable as it is difficult to simulate a condition with acupuncture where some patients are getting sham treatment. In studies of acupuncture in other diseases with a sham group, no difference was seen between those randomized to active treatment versus sham treatment.

Thus far, only one nonblinded, pilot trial of acupuncture in PD has been published (7–8). This study looked at the safety and efficacy of acupuncture in 20 PWPs. While 85% of the patients reported subjective improvement of symptoms after treatment, qualitative measures did not show significant improvement except in the areas of sleep and rest. Nonetheless, no significant serious adverse events were reported. Therefore, to date, there remains insufficient scientific evidence to routinely recommend the use of acupuncture to treat PD. Moreover, acupuncture is generally not covered by insurance and usually requires multiple treatments.

What about massage therapy? Is massage good for me?

Massage therapy involves manipulation of muscles and other soft tissues of the body. Varieties of massage techniques range from gentle stroking and kneading of muscles to manual "deep tissue" massage (2). Types of massage include aromatherapy, craniofacial, lymphatic, myofascial, reflexology (which involves "reflex areas" mainly involving the feet, but occasionally the hands), rolfing (a technique of loosening and balancing connective tissues introduced by Dr. Ida Loft), shiatsu (a massage popularized by the Japanese based on finger pressure), sports, Swedish (a massage technique that copies the moves of gymnasts), and trigger point.

Anecdotal patient reports indicate that massage may provide relief in stiffness and muscle aches common in PD. Similar to acupuncture, there is no scientific evidence to support benefits of routine massage therapy for PD. It is usually not covered by insurance and requires multiple treatments.

Everyone in our support group is enrolled in a tai chi class. Is this real or hype?

Tai chi can be thought of as a combination of a moving form of yoga and meditation. The movements are performed slowly and gracefully with smooth and even transitions between each motion. Therefore, learning to perform the movements involves balance, alignment, fine motor control, and rhythm of movement. Proponents of tai chi believe that it improves walking, running, and, more importantly, balance. Many practitioners notice benefits in postural alignment. The meditative nature of the exercises is calming and relaxing. However, there is little scientific evidence supporting the practice of tai chi in improving symptoms of PD. Research has been underway in some centers looking for quantitative evidence of its benefit in PD.

What about exercise in PD?

With or without PD, the benefits of exercise have been consistently proven. Moderate to vigorous exercise is good for the heart; it helps control blood pressure, lowers the "bad cholesterol," and lessens the likelihood of developing strokes and heart attacks. At least 30 to 45 minutes of aerobic exercise for most days of the week is recommended by the American Heart Association. If you have a pedometer, 10,000 steps per day are recommended for a healthy living.

In PD, the disease-modifying effect of exercise has been shown in animal models. Rats who were subjected to regular physical activity did better with their artificially induced parkinsonism than those who were sedentary. In human epidemiological studies, PWPs who exercised regularly did better than those who did not.

Walking is the simplest form of exercise. Try to walk close to a mile (or more) each day, if you can. We also encourage exercises that promote symmetry, such as swimming. Since PD is often an asymmetrical illness affecting one side more than the other, swimming will force the arms in your "bad side" to swing and propel as well as the arm on your good side. Any aerobic exercise seems to be beneficial.

Other than consistency and symmetry, the most important thing to remember about exercise is safety. All the benefits are negated if one falls and sustains a hip fracture. Therefore, walking is only good if one has a reasonably low risk of tripping or falling. Biking is good if one can keep his or her balance, otherwise, a stationary bike will achieve the same effect. Many PWPs choose stationary bikes with seats that have backs on them to prevent falls.

Are dietary supplements safe in PD?

The National Institutes of Health (NIH) Office of Dietary Supplements defines a dietary supplement as a product that

- is intended to supplement the diet;
- contains one or more dietary ingredients (including vitamins, minerals, herbs or other botanicals, amino acids, and other substances) or their constituents;
- is intended to be taken by mouth as a pill, capsule, tablet, or liquid;
- is labeled on the front panel as being a *dietary supplement.*

The Office of Dietary Supplements cautions that published analyses of herbal supplements have found differences between ingredients listed on the label and the bottle's actual ingredients. The word "standardized" on a product label is not a guarantee of higher product quality, since in the United States there is no legal definition of standardized (or "certified" or "verified") supplements. Without further testing in a rigorous manner, there is little scientific evidence to support most of the substances that are marked for the treatment of PD.

Should I be taking coenzyme Q10?

Coenzyme Q10 is an antioxidant and a component of the energy-producing electron transport chain of mitochondria (the "powerhouse" of the cell). CoQ10 stabilizes and promotes the "complex I" in a chain of events that occur inside the mitochondria that ultimately leads to energy production. Complex I activity has been found to be abnormal in PD. Therefore, CoQ10 might play a role in correcting this deficiency. It is currently being investigated as a neuroprotective agent.

In a preliminary, double-blind placebo-controlled study in PD, patients who received high doses of coenzyme Q10 (those that took 1200 mg per day) were associated with a reduced rate of deterioration in motor function (based on a Parkinson scale) over 16 months (9). This result should be considered preliminary. We do know that the supplement is generally well tolerated in this disease population. The tested formulations have usually included vitamin E. Because the available results are still preliminary, and the supplement (especially at high doses) can get really expensive, we do not routinely recommend the use of CoQ10 for PD. Large-scale trials are now under way to determine if CoQ10 can slow the progression of PD.

Where are we on creatine? Can I now take it or should I wait further?

Creatine is a dietary supplement that has generally been used for improving performance in athletes. No major safety or tolerability problems have been noted with oral supplementation of creatine in doses as high as 20 grams per day for short periods. Just like CoQ10, creatine plays an important role in mitochondrial energy production, and there is evidence of mitochondrial dysfunction in PDs, in particular with deficits in complex I activity, where creatine and CoQ10 both play a crucial role.

To test whether creatine alters the course of early PD, a "futility" study was performed. Futility studies are a quicker way of finding out whether a drug is worth pursuing further or not. These studies use a smaller number of patients by comparing how a drug performs to a predetermined "historical control" rather than an actual placebo arm. This study showed that after 12 months of therapy among 200 PWPs with early disease who were randomized into three arms (creatine, minocycline, and placebo), the patients who received creatine on average worsened (in Parkinson scale points) by 5.6 points, those who received minocycline worsened by 7.1 points, and those who received placebo worsened by 8.4 points. Therefore, since PD is a progressive illness that is expected to gradually worsen over time, those who received creatine had the least amount of decline. Tolerability was 91% in the creatine group and 77% in the minocycline group (10). Because of these preliminary results, the scientific community is now embarking on a large-scale clinical trial, enrolling over 1,700+ PWPs to determine if, indeed, creatine can slow disease progression. Over 60 Parkinson clinical trial centers throughout North America have joined forces for this massive undertaking.

Is there really no role for vitamin E in PD?

Vitamin E is another antioxidant. Earlier observational studies suggested that vitamin E may have had a neuroprotective effect and may have decreased the risk of PD. Zhang and coworkers (11) evaluated the incidence of PD in two large cohorts of men and women who completed detailed and validated semiquantitative food frequency questionnaires. In this survey of thousands of volunteers, a total of 371 incident PD cases were identified from the Nurses' Health Study and the Health Professionals Follow-Up Study. Neither intake of total vitamins E or C nor use of vitamin E or vitamin C supplements or multivitamins was associated with decreased risk of developing PD. The risk of PD, however, was reduced among men and women with high intake of dietary vitamin E from foods only.

The DATATOP study (12) found that vitamin E in doses of 2000 IU, did not delay the need for levodopa treatment among early PWPs. Furthermore, a grouped-analysis by Miller and coworkers (13) of 19 different clinical trials on vitamin E found that high dosage of vitamin E supplementation at 400 IU per day for a minimum of 1 year increased mortality. The benefits and risks of lower-dosage vitamin E supplementation were unclear.

Therefore, given the negative results of vitamin E in Parkinson's trials, and the potential for increased mortality with high doses, we do not recommend the use of vitamin E for the purpose of slowing the progression of PD.

What's the deal with glutathione?

The use of glutathione is a hot and controversial issue in PD because some patients and clinicians who administer the treatment really believe in its benefit. However, the drug is given intravenously and over time its cumulative cost can be really expensive. Glutathione is yet another anti-oxidant and also an essential "cofactor" for antioxidant enzymes. It provides protection for the mitochondria against harmful oxygen radicals (14). Several studies have demonstrated a deficiency of glutathione in the substantia nigra (the area of the brain affected in PD) of patients. However, it is not well absorbed in an oral formulation, so it is often given intravenously.

In a small, open-label study that looked at the effects of glutathione in nine patients with early, untreated PD (15) glutathione was administered intravenously, 600 mg twice daily for 30 days. All patients were reported to improve significantly after glutathione therapy, with a 42% decline in their disability. Once glutathione was stopped, the therapeutic effect lasted for an extra 2 to 4 months. However, there are still no published double-blind, placebo-controlled clinical trials on glutathione in PD. A pilot, double-blind, placebo-controlled study has just been completed at the University of South Florida. We should know the results very soon, but currently do not recommend glutathione in PD.

What other alternative treatments have been tried by PWPs?

Dehydroepiandrosterone (DHEA) is a hormone produced by the body (termed *endogenous* hormone). DHEA levels in the body normally begin to decline after age 30. DHEA can raise the levels of androgens and estrogens in the body and theoretically may increase the risk of prostate, breast, ovarian, and other hormone-sensitive cancers. DHEA has been investigated because some research suggests that increasing estrogen may be beneficial, if not potentially neuroprotective, in PD (16). For example, in an epidemiological study involving over 10,000 Parkinson residents in a nursing home, those who were on estrogen replacement therapy were found to be healthier, happier, and mentally sharper than those who were not on hormone replacement (17). However, while epidemiological studies (no matter how large they are) give us a clue of the possible benefit (or harm) of a substance, they are not "controlled" and "blinded" studies and are generally not considered as definitive evidence. Therefore, the estrogen (and DHEA) hypothesis has yet to be proven in PD.

Curcumin is another antioxidant that is derived from the curry spice turmeric. It may be an inducer of the "heat shock response" and has been hypothesized to reduce oxidative damage and amyloid pathology (the pathology seen in AD). There are no systematically derived human data available on curcumin for treatment of PD.

Enhanced external counterpulsation (EECP) is the sequential diastolic inflation of lower extremity pneumatic cuffs to augment aortic diastolic pressure, increase venous return to the heart, and decrease left ventricular "afterload." It is actually an approved treatment for angina. There have been websites that began offering EECP as a treatment for PD. The treatments are prescribed for one hour per day, five days a week, for six weeks. No scientific evidence supports its use. It is not covered by insurance and requires multiple treatments.

What about hair analysis and chelation therapy?

There are several websites offering hair analysis as a way of diagnosing heavy metal exposure (18). However, scientific studies demonstrate that this method is very unreliable, since external contaminants such as dust, shampoo, conditioners, or hair spray influence the results (19). Frequently, the results support the need for additional treatment such as chelation therapy.

Chelation therapy attempts to remove heavy metals from the body (20). Side effects may include fever, headache, nausea, vomiting, a sudden drop in blood pressure, abnormally low calcium levels in the blood, kidney damage, and bone marrow depression (damage to the "precursors" of red and white blood cells, compromising the body's ability to fight infection). There is no scientific evidence to support their use in PD. Moreover, even if certain heavy metals have been found to be elevated in individual patients, it is difficult to determine if this is directly due to PD, and there is no proof that removing the excess heavy metal will improve symptoms of PD.

What kind of treatments can improve my voice and communication? My friends and family can barely hear or understand me.

Of all speech therapy techniques, Lee Silverman Voice Therapy (LSVT) has the largest body of literature supporting its beneficial effects and is a popular treatment choice among PWPs with a soft voice and slurred speech (21). LSVT emphasizes phonatory effort and uses maximum performance tasks as the basis of intervention. LSVT also "recalibrates" an individual's perceived level of effort with an emphasis on self-awareness. Intact cognition is, therefore, a good prognostic indicator of success. However, LSVT can also be beneficial for patients with cognitive deficits.

Other treatments that may be appropriate include rate control techniques and the use of delayed auditory feedback

Augmentative-alternative communication (AAC) treatment approaches may also be beneficial in PD, particularly as the speech impairment worsens (22).

- Voice amplifiers may increase the volume of speech.
- Pacing boards may assist in rate control.

- Alphabet boards may be an effective strategy to supplement speech and provide context for communication partners.
- Other AAC strategies such as communication boards/notebooks, voice output computer systems, and portable typing devices may be used.

What treatments can alleviate swallowing problems in PD?

Interestingly, the LSVT, commonly used to improve speech in individuals with PD, was potentially effective for treatment for swallowing problems in a small number of patients. Recent research by Christine Sapienza at the University of Florida has shown that expiratory muscle strength training (EMST), using a small calibrated device that you blow into, may be the best available technique to improve swallowing. The EMST device is now available for purchase and there are ongoing studies to determine its optimal use in PD. In addition, beneficial techniques and postures can be implemented in a treatment program. Smaller, more frequent meals may be valuable to satisfy nutritional requirements while optimizing swallowing function, especially if swallowing is effortful or causes fatigue (23). Referral to an occupational therapist may also be beneficial to determine the usefulness of adaptive utensils and equipment in promoting independence with meals.

What assistive devices and "home remedies" can improve the activities of daily living of a PWP?

Assistive devices are sometimes recommended to sustain the patient's independence in their care and to increase their safety during their performance of tasks. During occupational therapy, the primary focus is the safe and optimal performance of tasks. Accommodation techniques are stressed. The patient and the caregiver are also instructed regarding environmental adaptations (24). Below is a list of the areas evaluated during occupational therapy and some examples of the strategies used.

- *Bed mobility*: teaching tricks of movement, using a ladder strap or a bed rail.
- *Mobility throughout the home*: rearranging the furniture, removal of throw rugs, reducing clutter or other pathway distractions, creating even lighting, using remote controls to operate the television or handheld phones to prevent rushing.
- *Showering*: using soap-on-a-rope, terry cloth robes for drying, and shower benches.

- *Toileting*: raising toilet seats and installing grab bars.
- *Grooming*: using electric shavers; teaching stabilization of the upper extremities on the edge of the sink to increase the stability of the arms for tasks.
- *Dressing*: teaching adaptive methods to maximize successful movement patterns; choosing loose clothing with easy fasteners to minimize the need for fine motor control.
- *Feeding*: using security grip–handled utensils; preparation of small portions and more frequent meals and longer meal times to prevent rushing.
- *Meal preparation*: using adaptive jar openers, rocker knives, or non-skid pads.
- *Household chores*: using lightweight vacuum cleaners and dust mop, using long-handled scrub brushes when the patient is unable to bend to reach the tub or overhead reach for ceiling fan blades.

How can I improve my handwriting?

Poor handwriting is one of the primary reasons for referral to an occupational therapist. Many PWPs have writing difficulties. These can include a lack of legibility because of the tremor, or writing really small letters (micrographia). Handwriting can negatively impact quality of life if it affects the patient's ability to sign a check, to make a note to their spouse, or to perform a task at work (24). Some nonpharmacological treatments of handwriting problems include the following:

- Exercises to increase in-hand manipulation skills
- Eye/hand coordination drills
- Provision of proximal stability
- Graded individual finger movement exercises
- Alternate methods with the use of a computer
- Creating a writing splint
- Enrolling in the Callirobics Writing Program

Are there certain diets that can help my swallowing problems?

Yes, usually a speech-language pathologist (SLP) can perform a swallowing evaluation with modified food consistency if needed. If the SLP determines thickened liquids or pureed foods are needed, you can then be referred to a registered dietician for nutrition assessment and appropriate diet planning.

My doctor says that I have a delay in the passage of food into my small intestines, she called it "gastroparesis." Is there anything I can do for this condition other than taking more pills?

Yes. Having numerous small meals and snacks instead of three large meals may help. Foods that are rich in nutrients and moderate in fat and fiber are preferred. Your protein needs should be assessed, and it should be divided equally among your meals. Your levodopa should be taken about 30 minutes before eating. You can supplement with low-protein snacks between these meals to meet your total calorie requirements. Occasionally, drugs such as erythromycin are helpful with gastric motility.

Please help me with my constipation.

Believe it or not, exercising helps quite a bit. Try to walk, move, and stretch daily. Consuming at least 25 grams of dietary sources of insoluble fiber, along with six- to eight-ounce glasses of fluids, will help to increase stool bulk and speed colon transit time. The use of both prebiotics (these are materials that promote the growth of beneficial microorganisms in the digestive system) and probiotics (these are dietary supplements containing beneficial bacteria or yeasts to the digestive system) may be helpful, along with servings of laxative foods such as prunes and kiwifruit. Your dietician can assess fiber and fluid intake and provide individualized counseling as needed. Diet and lifestyle changes should always be the preferred method of managing constipation for as long as possible, to avoid chronic laxative use.

What types of psychological support are available for PWPs?

Providing psychosocial evaluation and treatment is an important component in the management of PWPs and their families. This care is best delivered by mental health professionals such as psychiatrists, clinical psychologists, psychotherapists, clinical social workers, psychiatric clinical nurse specialists, and psychiatric nurses.

Possible interventions include psychotherapy, relaxation therapy, biofeedback, patient/family counseling, and support group facilitation. These interventions can help common problems in PD such as anxiety, depression, apathy, compulsive disorders, psychosis, dementia, alteration in family processes, social isolation, and alteration in role performance.

How can I get a good night's sleep "the natural way"? I would like to avoid taking sleeping pills if I can help it.

Getting a good night's sleep is important so that you feel rested the next day. Sometimes, severe motor fluctuations during the day is a result of poor sleep at night. Here are a few tips you can try (25):

- Maintain a regular sleep schedule seven days a week. Keep the same bedtime each night and take bedtime medications at the same time each evening.
- Make the sleep environment as comfortable as possible. Consider a bed with capability to elevate your head. Use satin sheets to move easier. Install a grab bar or mobility transfer handle to assist you with turning and getting in and out of bed. Have a comfortable recliner chair in room. And keep your bedroom clear of clutter.
- Avoid stimulants including caffeine, nicotine, and alcohol too close to bedtime.
- Participate in an active exercise program during the day.
- Spend part of the day outdoors, increasing natural exposure to light.
- If you take naps, take them early and for no longer than an hour.
- Avoid heavy meals within four hours of bedtime.
- Limit fluid intake four hours before bedtime.

Also, it is actually best to also avoid alcohol at night. It may seem like alcohol is a good sedative, but it can disrupt the rest of the sleep cycle.

Table 6.1 lists nonpharmacological approaches to the various sleep disturbances in PD.

Table 6.1 Nonpharmacological Approaches to Sleep Disturbances in Parkinson's Disease

Sleep disturbance	Nonpharmacological management
Nocturnal motor symptoms (dystonia, rigidity)	Reduce nightly dose of dopaminergic medications (for nocturnal dyskinesias)
Restless legs syndrome	Iron supplementation
	Folate
Rapid eye movement sleep behavior disorder	Ensure safety of sleep environment for patient and spouse
Excessive daytime sleepiness	Scheduled naps
	Exercise
Obstructive sleep apnea	Weight loss
Depression	Cognitive behavioral therapy
Frequent urination at night	Restrict fluids before bedtime
	Bedside commode
Hallucinations	Decrease dopaminergic medications
Primary insomnia	Review good sleep hygiene

Source: Adapted from Ref. 26.

What nonpharmacological treatments are available for autonomic problems in PD?

Table 6.2 lists some of the nonpharmacological remedies for some of the autonomic problems frequently encountered in PD.

When should I start looking for an alternative care setting for my husband with PD? He refuses to move to a nursing home and I am trying my best to support him.

PD is a chronic, progressive disorder, and care for individuals with this illness exists on a continuum (25). Not everyone needs to move to a nursing home, but when daily care becomes challenging, you have several alternatives.

Table 6.2 Nonpharmacologic Remedies for Autonomic Disturbances in Parkinson's Disease

Symptom	Nonpharmacological management
Orthostatic hypotension (sudden drop in blood pressure when standing)	Taper or discontinue unnecessary drugs that lower blood pressure (such as antihypertensives)
	Elevate head of bed 10–30 degrees
	Increase dietary salt (add salt tablets)
	Thigh-high, fitted compression stockings
	Education: avoid standing quickly, hot environment, straining-type exercises, etc.
Constipation	Add dietary bulk
	Increase fluid intake
	Regular exercise
	Mineral/tap water enemas
Excessive drooling	Encourage voluntary swallowing of saliva
	Sugar-free gum/hard candy
Erectile dysfunction	Eliminate drugs that cause this side effect
	Take it "easy and slow." Find creative ways of showing love and providing pleasure to your partner to take off the pressure of "performing."
Urinary frequency (hyperactive bladder)	Limit fluid intake 4 hours before bedtime
	Consider a condom catheter, or bedside commode
Urinary retention (hypoactive bladder)	Limit fluid intake 4 hours before bedtime
	Consider intermittent self-catheterization
Drenching sweats/diaphoresis	Prevent wearing off symptoms at night
	Wear loose cotton shirts

Source: Adapted from Ref. 26.

Adult day health programs exist throughout the United States to provide a supportive environment for individuals who are unable to safely or socially remain at home during daytime hours. These settings are designed for patients to participate in community life through a variety of programs and with individuals who share common interests and needs. Licensed health care professionals are on site to provide close supervision, medical monitoring, and medication management.

Individuals with PD utilize adult day health programs for a variety of reasons, including increased need for socialization, assistance with management of complex medication schedules, assistance with mobility due to fluctuations in motor response, safety monitoring due to an increased risk of falls, assistance with activities of daily living, and respite for family caregivers. Additional information on adult day health programs can be obtained by visiting the website of the National Adult Day Services Association (www.nadsa.org).

Assisted living communities provide homelike setting designed typically for seniors who are no longer able, for a wide variety of reasons, to live independently but do not require the level of care provided in a nursing home. Services include assistance with activities of daily living and management of medications, which are essential for individuals affected by PD. Most communities provide licensed nursing and rehabilitation services. Other beneficial outreach includes recreational and social programs, exercise and fitness classes, and in some circumstances, on-site PD support groups.

Useful resources about these communities for health care providers to assist patients and families include National Center for Assisted Living (www.ncal.org), American Assisted Living Nurses Association (www.alnursing.org), American Association of Homes and Services for the Aging (www.aahsa.org), Long Term Care Living (www.longtermcareliving.com), and A Place for Mom (www.aplaceformom.com).

Home care is provided for individuals with PD by primary and secondary caregivers. Primary caregivers are generally family members, usually a spouse or close friends. Secondary caregivers include individuals who provide skilled care such as licensed nurses, physical therapists, occupational therapists, SLPs, social workers, and home health aides. In addition, there are those who provide nonskilled care. These are homemakers and personal care attendants.

Home health care agencies exist to provide comprehensive home care services. They may be for-profit, nonprofit, or governmental. The programs may provide skilled services or nonskilled services or both.

Skilled services may be reimbursable by insurance coverage for a certain period of time. Nonskilled services are reimbursed only by certain long-term care insurances and private pay. Referrals for skilled services can be made from the short-term rehabilitation facility by the discharge planners or directly from a patient's physician. Certain criteria exists to receive reimbursable skilled home care including having a certain period of being homebound.

Do I need to join a Parkinson's "support group"?

Support groups exist all over the world to help PWPs and their family members better cope with this chronic condition. The meetings become a vehicle for providing education, socialization, coping strategies, and mutual support. Most groups follow a "self-help" model. This means they are member run and are composed of individuals who share the same situation. Some groups will share facilitator duties with a health care professional, most often a social worker or nurse. There are limited studies of the benefits of PD support groups; however, their increasing numbers and the widespread participation attest to the importance of their existence.

Each person is different. Choosing whether and when to join a support group is an important decision for a patient and family. Each group's function is uniquely dependent on a number of factors: group location, age of the members, years in existence, and group leadership, to name a few. Just as with anything, what works for one person may not work for another. The worst thing you can do as a patient joining a support group is getting discouraged when you see other people worse than you, thinking that you will one day be like them. Remember, PD is a very individual disorder. Each patient has his or her own course. The most ideal support group participant is someone who derives inspiration from other patients doing better, and who serves as an inspiration to the rest of the members in the group doing worse.

If you have the right attitude, it is great to be part of a support group. Knowledge is power. There is only so much your doctor or nurse practitioner can tell you in a 30-minute office visit. The rest you will need to read and learn on your own. There is not a better way to educate yourself than learning from other's successes and failures.

Recently, many support groups have evolved to serve specific subgroups, such as young-onset PD.

FURTHER READING

Etminan M, Gill SS, Samii A. Intake of vitamin E, vitamin C, and carotenoids and the risk of Parkinson's disease: a meta-analysis. *Lancet Neurol.* 2005;4(6):362–365.

Jenner P. Oxidative damage in neurodegenerative disease. *Lancet.* 1994;796–798.

Yorkston KM, Beukelman DR, Strand EA, Bell KR. *Management of Motor Speech Disorders in Children and Adults.* Austin, TX: Pro-Ed; 1999.

REFERENCES

1. Rajedran PR, Thompson RE, Reich SG. The use of alternative therapies by patients with Parkinson's disease. *Neurology.* 2001;57:790–794.

2. Mclain T, Hauser RA. Complementary therapies in Parkinson's disease. In: Grosset DG, Grosset KA, Okun MS, Fernandez HH, eds. *Clinician's Desk Reference: Parkinson's Disease.* London: Manson; 2009.

3. Forrelli T. Understanding herb-drug interactions. *Techniques in Orthopaedics.* 2003;18(1):37–45.

4. Hu Z, Yang X, Ho P, et al. Drug interactions: a literature review. *Drugs.* 2005;65(9):1239–1282.

5. Manyam BV, Sanchez-Ramos JR. Traditional and complementary therapies in Parkinson's disease. *Adv Neurol.* 1999;80:565–574.

6. Katzenschlager R, Evans A, Manson A, et al. Mucuna pruriens in Parkinson's disease: a double blind clinical and pharmacological study. *J Neurol Neurosurg Psychiatry.* 2004;75(12):1672–1677.

7. Rabinstein A, Shulman L. Acupuncture in clinical neurology. *Neurologist.* 2003;9(3):137–148.

8. Shulman LM, Wen X, Weiner WJ, et al. Acupuncture therapy for the symptoms of Parkinson's disease. *Mov Disord.* 2002;17:799–802.

9. Shults CW, Oakes D, Kieburtz K, et al. Effects of coenzyme Q10 in early Parkinson disease: evidence of slowing of the functional decline. *Arch Neurol.* 2002;59(10):1541–1550.

10. NINDS NET-PD Investigators. A pilot clinical trial of creatine and minocyclinie in early Parkinson disease: 18 month results. *Clin Neuropharmacol.* 2008;31(3):141–150.

11. Zhang SM, Hernan MA, Chen H, Spiegelman D, Willett WC, Ascherio A. Intakes of vitamins E and C, carotenoids, vitamin supplements, and PD risk. Comments. *Neurology.* 2002;59(8):E8–E9.

12. Parkinson Study Group. Effects of tocopherol and deprenyl on the progression of disability in early Parkinson's disease. *N Engl J Med.* 1993;328:176–183.

13. Miller ER, Pastor-Barriuso R, Dalal D, Riemersma RA, Appel LJ, Guallar E. Meta-analysis: high-dosage vitamin E supplementation may increase all-cause mortality. *Ann Intern Med.* 2005;142(1):37–46.

14. Adams JD Jr, Klaidman LK, Odunze IN, Shen HC, Miller CA. Alzheimer's and Parkinson's disease. Brain levels of glutathione, glutathione disulfide, and vitamin E. *Mol Clin Neuropathol.* 1991;14:213–226.

15. Sechi G, Deledda MG, Bua G, et al. Reduced intravenous glutathione in the treatment of early Parkinson's disease. *Progress in Neuro-Psychopharmacology & Biol Psychiatry.* 196;20(7):1159–1170.

16. Cyr M, Calon F, Morissette M, Grandbois M, Di Paolo T, Callier S. Drugs with estrogen-like potency and brain activity: potential therapeutic application for the CNS. *Curr Pharm Des.* 2000;6(12):1287–1312.

17. Fernandez HH, Lapane KL; for the SAGE (Systematic Assessment of Geriatric Drug use via Epidemiology) Study Group. Estrogen use among nursing home residents with a diagnosis of Parkinson's disease. *Mov Disord.* 2000;15:1119–1124.

18. Barrett S. Commercial hair analysis: a cardinal sign of quackery. 8http://www.quackwatch.com/01Quackery RelatedTopics/hair.html. Cited January 2, 2005.

19. Seidel S, Kreutzer R, Smith D, McNeel S, Gilliss D. Assessment of commercial laboratories performing hair mineral analysis. *JAMA.* 2001;285:67–72.

20. Frumkin H, Manning CC, Williams PL, et al. Diagnostic chelation challenge with DMSA: a biomarker of long-term mercury exposure? *Environ Health Perspect.* 2001;109:167–171.

21. Ramig LO, Brin MF, Velickovic M, Fox C. Hypokinetic laryngeal movement disorders. In: Kent RD, ed. *The MIT Encyclopedia of Communication Disorders.* Cambridge, MA: The MIT Press; 2004:30–32.

22. Beukelman DR, Yorkston KM, Reichle J. *Augmentative and Alternative Communication for Adults With Acquired Neurologic Disorders.* Baltimore, MD: Paul H. Brookes; 2000.

23. Yorkston KM, Miller RM, Strand EA. *Management of Speech and Swallowing in Degenerative Diseases.* San Antonio, TX: Communication Skill Builders; 1995.

24. Myers KJ, Gardner-Smith P. Role of the physical and occupational therapist. In: Grosset DG, Grosset KA, Okun MS, Fernandez HH, eds. *Clinician's Desk Reference: Parkinson's Disease.* London: Mansion; 2008.

25. Tuite PJ, Thomas CA, Rukert LF, Fernandez HH. *Parkinson's Disease: A Guide to Patient Care.* New York, NY: Springer. In press.

26. Kluger BM, Fernandez HH. Management of non-motor manifestations of Parkinson's disease. In: Simuni T, Pahwa R, eds. *Parkinson's Disease.* New York, NY: Oxford University Press; 2009:83–94.

My 85-year-old mom has had Parkinson's disease for 30 years and is currently on Sinemet (25/100 mg) every 2 hours and 75 mg of quetiapine at bedtime.

She has extreme difficulty forming words with her lips. We cannot understand what she is trying to say. Her speech volume is very low. Are speech volume and inability to form words both symptoms of Parkinson's disease? Is there anyone we should see who can help her? Thank you.

CHAPTER 7

Multidisciplinary Approaches to Treatment

What is the difference between a multidisciplinary approach to Parkinson's treatment and an interdisciplinary approach and why does it matter?

Most medical offices offer simple old-fashioned medicine. You simply make an appointment, visit the doctor, undergo an examination, obtain a prescription (if warranted), and then return in a few weeks or months for a checkup. PD care is, however, much better when administered in a multi/interdisciplinary environment (1–5). A multidisciplinary practice offers an organized referral service for multiple specialties (eg, physical therapy, occupational therapy speech, psychology, etc.). In addition, specialists can speak to one another through letters, notes, and telephone correspondence. In an interdisciplinary approach, all the members of the case team are usually present and meet to discuss your care. The latter, interdisciplinary approach is therefore better than a multidisciplinary evaluation when it is available (6). Unfortunately, due to the economic environment and the current restraints of the US health care systems most doctors and clinics cannot afford a multi/interdisciplinary approach. There are funding agencies, such as the NPF, who have championed this approach both by funding centers of excellence and also by training multi/interdisciplinary teams (NPF's allied team training for PD). A recent Canadian study led by Mark Guttman, MD, at the NPF Center of Excellence in Markam, Ontario (presented at the International Congress of Movement Disorders in Istanbul, Turkey), revealed the superiority of a multi/interdisciplinary approach to care.

What is the role of the movement disorders neurologist, and does my neurologist need special training in PD?

A general neurologist in the United States must complete a four-year accredited neurology residency (1 year of internal/general medicine and 3 years of neurology). You may be surprised to learn that a very large percentage of general neurologists have not passed their neurology boards (a good question that patients seldom inquire about). A general neurologist is trained to deal with all neurological maladies, and most do not have much training beyond the core principles of diagnosis of PD. Making the situation worse, many neurology residents receive little to no instruction on the care of the PWP within the outpatient setting. This situation translates in practice to mean that patients seeking excellent PD care should seek either physicians with some interest in PD, physicians who have dedicated most of their practice to PWPs, or a physician who has completed postresidency fellowship training in PD and movement disorders. Moreover, the patient and family should inquire as to whether that physician is linked to a complete complement of multi/interdisciplinary services, and/or to a peer-reviewed center of excellence. Since movement disorders neurologists and even neurologists with special interest in movement disorders are somewhat rare, patients may choose to travel once or twice a year to the nearest specialist, who in many cases is located within a university setting. The patient and family should advocate for the specialist to coordinate local care through a local neurologist. In this way, the patient wins, as they get local and specialized care, and the physicians win as they get to share a better managed and happier patient and family.

What is the role of the neuropsychologist and neuropsychological testing?

The neuropsychologist in PD care can play a vital role in the diagnosis and the management of a patient. Since the nonmotor symptoms of PD have such a high impact on the quality of life, a heavy value should be placed on psychology (7,8).

A neuropsychologist is a professional trained in examining all of the lobes (lobes are different brain regions) of the brain with written and oral (speaking) tests in order to offer diagnoses, follow the clinical course of disease, and recommend pharmacological and behavioral interventions. Neuropsychologists will often diagnose and work with physicians on a treatment plan for affective and mental illnesses.

A counseling psychologist, who is also an important part of the team, regularly meets with patients offering cognitive behavioral therapies (these therapies are talking therapies given over several appointments with the counseling psychologist) and also support therapies to treat mental and neurological illness.

Both counseling psychologists and neuropsychologists work with patients and families to enhance overall care and care delivery.

PWPs almost always have problems with the frontal lobes of the brain (they are in charge of initiating and inhibiting behavior) and problems with memory. There are many things psychologists can offer to help patients, and one active area of research interest has been the development of cognitive rehabilitation strategies (9,10).

The neuropsychologist may play a major role in the evaluation for the appropriateness of DBS therapy. DBS presents a host of unique opportunities—and challenges—for mental health professionals. Psychological issues may be highly relevant to the success of DBS treatment. There are important roles for mental health professionals both before and after DBS surgery. Note that there may also be opportunities for mental health professionals to assist intraoperatively, including administration of relaxation exercises and/or guided visual imagery immediately before, during, or following DBS-related procedures (eg, lead implantation, programming) (11,12).

What is the role of the psychiatrist in the PD team?

"Screening for disturbances of mood and perception comprise an integral part of the assessment of a patient with Parkinson's disease. Disturbances in mood may be widely variable and for example range from adjustment disorders, to major depression, and even mania. Disturbances in perception also occur in Parkinson's disease and range from subtle delusional states to frank hallucinations. Additionally there must be an assessment of anxiety symptoms and this may yield treatable conditions such as obsessions, compulsions, excessive worry or panic attacks. It is important to have a comprehensive psychiatric evaluation in all Parkinson's disease patients. Quality of life and overall treatment success may hinge on recognition of and appreciation for psychiatric illness in this challenging patient group. There is a large potential role for the psychiatrist on the multi/interdisciplinary care team" (13).

It has been estimated that depressive symptoms are common in all disorders that involve a group of brain circuits called the basal ganglia (14). Depressive symptoms occur in a majority of PWPs and seem to be the result of deficiencies in multiple brain chemicals (15,16). They are treatable, and for this reason, depression and other psychiatric comorbidities should be sought and aggressively treated in PD.

What is the role of the physical therapist in the PD team?

"Physical therapy can offer opportunity for those living with Parkinson's disease. Parkinson's disease presents in a variety of forms and therapists should be aware that it can affect mobility, posture, balance, and therefore impact an individual's ability to perform everyday tasks. Physical therapy does not necessarily address the underlying Parkinson's disease mechanism, but rather focuses on treating symptoms and secondary conditions that may accompany the Parkinson's disease phenomena. Through the management of these secondary conditions, therapists can create a foundation to maintain and improve function for select patients. The physical therapist may employ various treatment modalities and provide guidance to help individuals recognize and manage compensatory movements, as well as habits that may have developed as a result of the Parkinson's disease. Making sufferers aware of activities that aggravate symptoms and teaching beneficial substitute methods may contribute to improved motor control and to quality of life. Physical therapy may also enhance the benefits from other medical treatments, such as oral medications, botulinum toxin injections and surgical interventions. Physical therapy is a slow process that should be approached with the expectation that there will be a significant commitment in time, but with that commitment should come optimism. Results may not be immediately apparent, but a physical therapy program can influence many aspects of daily living, and also prevention of falling, improvements in balance, and the selection of appropriate assistive devices" (17). Physical therapy may be needed throughout the course of PD multi/interdisciplinary care, and it should be adapted or tailored to the patient's needs as conditions change and especially as symptoms may become resistant to levodopa. Physical therapy, exercise therapy, treadmill training, tai chi, and other alternative therapies may all have a role in improving the symptoms of PD (18–29).

What is the role of the occupational therapist in the PD team?

"The occupational therapist has a unique and compelling role in the evaluation and treatment of individuals with PD. Occupational therapy is an applied science and rehabilitation profession aimed at enabling individuals to reach their maximum potential in performance of daily living skills, in work and school productivity, and in leisure, through the use of purposeful activity. Occupational therapy uses purposeful, therapeutic activities to prevent and mediate dysfunction, and to promote adaptation in an individual. The ultimate goal of the treatment program is to restore the individual to their maximum level of performance in valued occupational roles through restorative or compensatory treatment approaches. Occupational therapists work with patients to help them to develop the skills and strategies to utilize mainly their hands and upper extremities in addressing real-life tasks (handwriting, eating, drinking, etc.). Occupational therapists work hand in hand with the other members of the multi/interdisciplinary team" (30).

What is the role of the social worker in the PD team?

"Social work has evolved to encompass a wide range of skills including biopsychosocial assessment, education, communication, advocacy, counseling, and case management. Each specific skill may offer a valuable perspective to the interdisciplinary/multidisciplinary team as well as to the patient, the family, and the patient's support system. The diagnosis of any serious, chronic illness may typically be associated with a constellation of psychosocial issues for the patient, family and caregivers. Some of these issues can present immediately at the time of diagnosis and continue throughout the illness while others may develop gradually over the duration of the illness. Some problems may resolve over a period of time. It is important that on a continuous basis social workers ask about and be aware of a patient's own assessment of their *current* experiences and feelings. With the consent of the patient, it is also important to ask family members and caregivers for an assessment of patient functioning. Patients may react to the news of a serious illness in various ways, and some reactions may be more constructive than others. Falvo has noted that in the care of patients, "how individuals view their condition, its causes and its consequences greatly affects what they do in the face of it" (31). Some patients express relief at finally hearing a diagnosis that may explain long-standing symptoms, however others may find the words devastating and immediately life altering. Others when confronted with bad news may react with denial. Whatever the initial reaction, suddenly having to face the management of any chronic illness often exposes the patient and family to multiple new stressors. This can include depression, grief, false hopes, financial pressures, the disruption of established family roles and difficulty adhering to complicated treatment regimens over a long term. All the above can put a great deal of strain on interpersonal relationships. For caregivers depression, fatigue and burnout are common risks. Ideally, the social worker is paired with the patient and the family as soon as possible following the diagnosis. In this situation it is useful to follow the patient's cues on the degree and frequency of support they desire. It may take a while for the patient to digest the information given to them. Initially, simply acknowledging the diagnosis may be a sufficient step toward coping. Other patients and families may want additional information right away about the diagnosis or how to access community resources or concrete services. The social worker must work in concert with the multi/interdisciplinary care team to tailor a treatment for individual patients and families" (32).

What is the role of the speech therapist/nutritionist in the PD team?

The speech and swallowing therapist, often referred to as a speech pathologist, has the important task of making sure that the PWP can communicate clearly and that swallowing disability is identified and rapidly treated. Again this clinician plays a key role on the team and ensures coordination of services between the multi/interdisciplinary specialties. Hypophonia or soft speech is often treated, and one common approach has been LSVTs. Coughing while eating may be a signal of swallowing problems, and there are many therapies including a new therapy called expiratory muscle strength training that may be employed. During the history, the speech clinician is able to observe connected speech while obtaining the necessary information. The clinician should pay attention to the use of any compensatory strategies. In some cases the speech therapist may offer exercises and techniques as well as changes in diet and food consistency. In other cases they may be involved in the multi/interdisciplinary decision for a feeding tube. The speech clinician must be aware how speech may change in different environments and during different tasks (eg, reading, singing, conversation), and they must obtain specific information regarding medical treatments (eg, botulinum toxin or surgical intervention) and their effect on speech.

Both the patient and family must provide the history that will guide diagnosis and treatment, and usually both must be involved in the long-term solution (33–41).

The speech therapist often works with a nutritionist to choose the best and safest diet for an individual PWP. A small minority of patients will have a problem where high protein diets interfere with absorption of dopamine tablets. In these cases taking medications one hour prior to eating or changing dietary protein content may be helpful. Finally, in the case where medications do not seem to be working, the nutritionist may recommend a gastric emptying study, as many PWPs have gastrointestinal dysfunction.

There is a new exciting therapy being developed at the University of Florida by Christine Sapienza to address aspiration and swallowing dysfunction. The therapy is called expiratory muscle strength training and is a simple device the patient may blow into to improve swallowing.

Preliminary results of trials sponsored by the Michael J. Fox Foundation (featured on Dateline NBC) and the NIH are due to be published soon.

What questions should I be asking when I come to clinic for an evaluation?

During your first clinic visit you should enquire as to the experience of the doctor and the staff. Do not be alarmed if the practice you are visiting utilizes nurses, nurse practitioners, or physician's assistants in *new* and *return* visits. Often these health care professionals are more on top of your care than your physician who may be very busy. Physicians who have completed fellowships beyond their neurology residency and those who are board certified are of course preferable; however, you must realize that there are very few movement disorders specialists worldwide. Many physicians have dedicated a large part of their practice to PD and movement disorders (>50%), and they may be able to provide you with spectacular care. It is best if you can coordinate visits to be shared between a local neurologist and a specialist (who may be at a distance from your home, eg, a university center).

Make sure you enquire as to how you can ask emergent, urgent, and routine questions once you have returned home following your visit. One issue that repeatedly comes up in PD care is access. Make sure the practice you have chosen has some sort of return telephone policy and a way to work in urgent appointments in a reasonable amount of time. You should ask the practice what you can do to help increase the efficiency of care (eg, will they allow you to use email or fax in your prescription refills?).

Finally, make sure there is access to information. Many offices have free patient education booklets, or they can point you toward resources that can update you on the latest developments in PD research. Many patients fail to ask the question at each visit: "is there something new out that may help my case of PD?" Make sure wherever you seek care they have a connection to the latest PD clinical trials and that they will grant you access to a multidisciplinary team of para-health professionals for all of your needs.

What information should I assemble prior to my appointment that will make my time more effective?

For new patient visits, the following information is useful and, when organized, will make your appointment smoother and of higher quality (you will have more time for questions and interactions rather than record review).

- A summary document that details in bullet points the main PD symptoms you have had since diagnosis (organized by year).
- A summary document that includes all of the medications and doses you have tried (organized by year), and also details about side effects or benefits with each.
- A complete list of your medical illnesses and past surgeries (organized by year).
- A list of your top five priorities or symptoms you would like addressed in this appointment.
- Finally under the summaries above, include copies of all your medical records and obtain the actual head and/or spine MRIs and CTs (most imaging facilities will burn these for you on a disk). The best neurologists will personally review your imaging rather than trusting reports.

For return visits, assemble the following information:

- A list of your current medications/doses (most PWPs like to use charts with the time at the top and the medications in a list along the left side).
- A bullet point summary (brief) of any changes or health problems since the last visit (clinic visits, hospitalizations, etc.)
- A list of your top five priorities or symptoms to be addressed in this appointment.
- If you have had any images of your brain or spine, bring the actual images for review (usually burned on a CD).

Below is a sample medication list as it is typically organized for new and return visits:

Medication and dose	8 AM	12 PM	4 PM	8 PM	11 PM
Sinemet 25/100	1	1	1	1	
Sinemet 50/200 CR					1
Mirapex 1 mg	1	1	1		
Rasagiline 1 mg	1				
Coenzyme Q10 400 mg	1	1	1		
Metopropol 20 mg	1				
Lipitor 20 mg	1				
Nexium 20 mg	1				

What does the term palliative therapy mean in PD?

The term palliative therapy has been defined by the National Cancer Institute to refer to "treatment given to relieve the symptoms and reduce the suffering caused by cancer and other life-threatening diseases. Palliative cancer therapies are given together with other cancer treatments, from the time of diagnosis, through treatment, survivorship, recurrent or advanced disease, and at the end of life." We often do not think of palliative care as part of PD, but in some sense we are neglecting our patients if we do not consider the aggressive treatment of the pain and suffering that may come along with chronic neurodegenerative diseases, particularly in those like PD with long disease durations.

Miyasaki and colleagues at the NPF Center of Excellence in Toronto have been studying palliative care. They have commented that "little is known about the lived health-care experiences of persons living with palliative stage Parkinson's disease and the family members who care for them." They conducted real patient interviews and discovered three main themes: "missing information, being on your own, wanting and not wanting to know." They concluded that palliative care needs are not being met in PD and that multidisciplinary teams should provide the comprehensive support. They are currently working on a program to implement these needs (42).

Similarly Goy and colleagues surveyed PWPs in Oregon and Washington about "symptoms, treatment preferences, health care usage, and psychosocial experiences during the last month of life." "Overall suffering in Parkinson's disease was rated at a median of 4 (1 = none to 6 = severe). Pain was moderately severe in 42% and the Parkinson's disease patients had confusion and significantly shorter hospice enrollments when compared to ALS patients (Lou Gehrig's disease)." These authors concluded that there needed to be studies to define hospice readiness and special needs in hospice that might improve end-of-life care for PWPs (43).

Why should I consider a feeding tube?

There are scenarios in a minority of PWPs where swallowing may become troublesome. Sometimes it is the PD itself, and other times there is a comorbid condition such as a small stroke or a diverticulum that may affect the ability to safely ingest food. The worry is that food may go down the air pipe (the trachea) and an aspiration pneumonia may result. One warning clue to swallowing dysfunction is the occurrence of cough during meals. PWPs with severe swallowing problems who may be at risk for aspiration often have good cognition and otherwise have an acceptable quality of life. Translated literally, unlike patients with more severe neurological syndromes, PWPs may actually have an enhancement in their quality of life with the placement of a feeding tube (called a percutaneous endoscopic gastrostomy [PEG] tube).

PWPs and their families should therefore not have an automatic allergy to the placement of a feeding tube. These days they can be placed by a radiologist or gastroenterologist and can be done with minimal risk and no need for an operating room. PWPs can sometimes even continue to eat through the mouth (safe foods cleared by a speech pathologist) and have the rest of their nutrition poured through the feeding tube. The tube can assist patients in feeling full, enhancing the quality of their life, and preventing wasting syndromes and weight loss.

Zelar and colleagues studied the long-term evolution of patients with neurological diseases after insertion of percutaneous endoscopic gastrostomy tubes. "PEG insertion was technically successful in all cases. The most frequent complications were minor and no aspiration pneumonias were reported." These authors suggested that PEG was the method of choice for enteral feeding of patients with chronic neurological disorders, and that PEG was well-tolerated, leading to an improvement in nutritional status" (44).

REFERENCES

1. Guttman M, Suchowersky O. Parkinson's disease management: towards a new paradigm. *Can J Neurol Sci.* 1999;26(suppl 2):S53–S57.
2. Playfer J. Targeting Parkinson's disease—the case for early referral. *Curr Med Res Opin.* 2000;16(1):43–45.
3. Carne W, Cifu D, Marcinko P, et al. Efficacy of a multidisciplinary treatment program on one-year outcomes of individuals with Parkinson's disease. *NeuroRehabilitation.* 2005;20(3):161–167.
4. Hagell P. Nursing and multidisciplinary interventions for Parkinson's disease: what is the evidence? *Parkinsonism Relat Disord.* 2007;13(suppl 3):S501–S508.
5. Visser M, van Rooden SM, Verbaan D, Marinus J, Stiggelbout AM, van Hilten JJ. A comprehensive model of health-related quality of life in Parkinson's disease. *J Neurol.* 2008;255(10):1580–1587.
6. Hagestuen R. Allied team training for Parkinson's disease. *NPF.* 2008.
7. Chaudhuri KR, Healy DG, Schapira AH. Non-motor symptoms of Parkinson's disease: diagnosis and management. *Lancet Neurol.* 2006;5(3):235–245.

8. Schrag A. Quality of life and depression in Parkinson's disease. *J Neurol Sci.* 2006;248(1–2):151–157.

9. McDougall GJ. Rehabilitation of memory and memory self-efficacy in cognitively impaired nursing home residents. *Clin Gerontol.* 2001;23(3–4):127–139.

10. Ball K, Berch DB, Helmers KF, et al. Effects of cognitive training interventions with older adults: a randomized controlled trial. *JAMA.* 2002;288(18):2271–2281.

11. Okun MS, Rodriguez RL, Mikos A, et al. Deep brain stimulation and the role of the neuropsychologist. *Clin Neuropsychol.* 2007;21(1):162–189.

12. Reckess G, Zahodne Z, Fenell E, Bowers D. The role of psychologist in dystonia. In: Okun MS, ed. *The Dystonia Patient: A Guide to Practical Management.* New York, NY: Demos; 2009.

13. Ward H. In: Okun MS, ed. *The Dystonia Patient: A Guide to Practical Management.* New York, NY: Demos; 2009.

14. Miller KM, Okun MS, Fernandez HF, Jacobson CE, Rodriguez RL, Bowers D. Depression symptoms in movement disorders: comparing Parkinson's disease, dystonia, and essential tremor. *Mov Disord.* 2007;22(5):666–672.

15. Aarsland D, Pedersen KF, Ehrt U, Bronnick K, Gjerstad MD, Larsen JP. Neuropsychiatric and cognitive symptoms in Parkinson disease [in Norwegian]. *Tidsskr Nor Laegeforen.* 2008;128(18):2072–2076.

16. Shutov AA, Dondova AI. Involvement of serotonergic system in the pathogenesis of non-motor symptoms of Parkinson's disease [in Russian]. *Zh Nevrol Psikhiatr Im S S Korsakova.* 2008;108(11):67–71.

17. Meyers K. *The Dystonia Patient: A Guide to Practical Management.* Demos; 2009.

18. Bloem BR, Boers I, et al. Falls in the elderly. I. Identification of risk factors [in German]. *Wien Klin Wochenschr.* 2001;113(10):352–362.

19. Bloem BR, Steijns JA, et al. An update on falls. *Curr Opin Neurol.* 2003;16(1):15–26.

20. Morris ME. Locomotor training in people with Parkinson disease. *Phys Ther.* 2006;86(10):1426–1435.

21. Suchowersky O, Reich S, et al. Practice parameter: diagnosis and prognosis of new onset Parkinson disease (an evidence-based review): report of the Quality Standards Subcommittee of the American Academy of Neurology. *Neurology.* 2006;66(7):968–975.

22. Ashburn A, Fazakarley L, et al. A randomised controlled trial of a home based exercise programme to reduce the risk of falling among people with Parkinson's disease. *J Neurol Neurosurg Psychiatry.* 2007;78(7):678–684.

23. Dennison AC, Noorigian JV, et al. Falling in Parkinson disease: identifying and prioritizing risk factors in recurrent fallers. *Am J Phys Med Rehabil.* 2007;86(8):621–632.

24. Gracies JM, Tse W, et al. Physical therapy in Parkinson's disease. *Handb Clin Neurol.* 2007;84:1–16.

25. Benatru I, Vaugoyeau M, et al. Postural disorders in Parkinson's disease. *Neurophysiol Clin.* 2008;38(6):459–465.

26. Dibble LE. It's not just about the score: using the full clinical picture to identify future fallers. *J Neurol Phys Ther.* 2008;32(3):148–149.

27. Goodwin VA, Richards SH, et al. The effectiveness of exercise interventions for people with Parkinson's disease: a systematic review and meta-analysis. *Mov Disord.* 2008;23(5):631–640.

28. Hackney ME, Earhart GM. Tai Chi improves balance and mobility in people with Parkinson disease. *Gait Posture.* 2008;28(3):456–460.

29. Kurtais Y, Kutlay S, et al. Does treadmill training improve lower-extremity tasks in Parkinson disease? A randomized controlled trial. *Clin J Sport Med.* 2008;18(3):289–291.

30. Gardner-Smith P. *The Dystonia Patient: A Guide to Practical Management.*New York, NY: Demos; 2009.

31. Falvo DR. *Medical and Psychosocial Aspects of Chronic Illness and Disability.* 3rd edn. 2005.

32. Greenhut G, McGhan G. *The Dystonia Patient: A Guide to Practical Management.* New York, NY: Demos; 2009.

33. Ramig LO, Countryman S, et al. Intensive speech treatment for patients with Parkinson's disease: short-and long-term comparison of two techniques. *Neurology.* 1996;47(6):1496–1504.

34. El Sharkawi A, Ramig L, et al. Swallowing and voice effects of Lee Silverman Voice Treatment (LSVT): a pilot study. *J Neurol Neurosurg Psychiatry.* 2002;72(1):31–36.

35. Ramig LO, Fox C, et al. Parkinson's disease: speech and voice disorders and their treatment with the Lee Silverman Voice Treatment. *Semin Speech Lang.* 2004;25(2):169–80.

36. Saleem AF, Sapienza CM, et al. Respiratory muscle strength training: treatment and response duration in a patient with early idiopathic Parkinson's disease. *NeuroRehabilitation.* 2005;20(4):323–333.

37. Fox CM, Ramig LO, et al. The science and practice of LSVT/LOUD: neural plasticity-principled approach to treating individuals with Parkinson disease and other neurological disorders. *Semin Speech Lang.* 2006;27(4):283–299.

38. Miller N, Noble E, et al. Hard to swallow: dysphagia in Parkinson's disease. *Age Ageing.* 2006;35(6):614–618.

39. Pitts T, Bolser D, et al. Impact of expiratory muscle strength training on voluntary cough and swallow function in Parkinson disease. *Chest.* 2008;

40. Troche MS, Sapienza CM, et al. Effects of bolus consistency on timing and safety of swallow in patients with Parkinson's disease. *Dysphagia.* 2008;23(1):26–32.

41. Plowman-Prine E, Jones H, Rosenbek J. *The Dystonia Patient: A Guide to Practical Management.* New York, NY: Demos; 2009.

42. Giles S, Miyasaki J. Palliative stage Parkinson's disease: patient and family experiences of health-care services. *Palliat Med.* 2008.

43. Goy ER, Carter J, et al. Neurologic disease at the end of life: caregiver descriptions of Parkinson disease and amyotrophic lateral sclerosis. *J Palliat Med.* 2008;11(4):548–554.

44. Zalar AE, Guedon C, et al. Percutaneous endoscopic gastrostomy in patients with neurological diseases. Results of a prospective multicenter and international study [in Spanish]. *Acta Gastroenterol Latinoam.* 2004;34(3):127–132.

I am 47 and have had Parkinson's disease for 10 years. I was approved for deep brain stimulation surgery and have undergone neuropsychological evaluation and received a call from the scheduling department indicating surgery has been approved. Ever since the approval, 10 days ago, my symptoms seem to be lessening. I only need the Sinemet three times daily. My rigidity, slowness, and tremor are not as significant. What could account for this? A placebo effect? I am now questioning the surgery even though I have been researching and deliberating for a year. Prior to the appointment with the neurosurgeon, two different movement disorder specialists suggested the surgery.

CHAPTER 8

Surgical Approaches to Treatment

What is DBS?

Deep brain stimulation (DBS) is a relatively new procedure that uses an implantable electrode, which may be used in place of or in conjunction with, other brain procedures such as pallidotomy or thalamotomy (where a portion of the brain is irreversibly burned) (1–5). PWPs and patients with tremor, dystonia, or OCD without Tourette's syndrome who are medically refractory to therapy and who have no cognitive difficulties or "minimal" cognitive (thinking issues) dysfunction may be appropriate candidates (6). There are also other expanding indications such as depression, cluster headache, and epilepsy (7–8).

The procedure is FDA approved for PD and the currently available technology is manufactured by the Medtronic corporation, although many companies are now involved in the development of brain hardware. The DBS lead has four electrode contacts (quadrapolar), and, depending on the disorder and/or the target, one may use variably sized contacts with different spacing arrangements. Each contact can be activated using monopolar (the current when passed to the brain is shaped like a big globe or sphere) or bipolar stimulation (the current when passed to the brain is shaped like an ellipse), and multiple settings can be adjusted for individual patient needs. The settings that may be adjusted include the pulse width (how big each pulse of stimulation is), frequency (how frequently per second we give each pulse), and amplitude of stimulation (how much voltage we pass through the lead). The DBS electrode is implanted into a specific target within the brain and is attached to a programmable pulse generator. The pulse generator is implanted in a pocket below the clavicle and connected to the DBS electrode in the brain. A tunneled extension

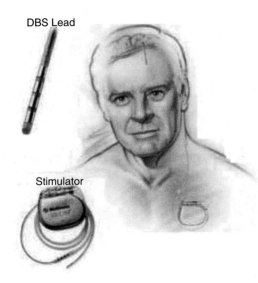

DBS Lead

Stimulator

Figure 8.1 Medtronic deep brain stimulator. (Courtesy of Medtronic Corporation, Minneapolis, MN).

cable then passes under the skin, over the clavicle, and across the posterior aspect of the neck and skull (the pulse generator is just like a cardiac pacemaker but the wire goes to the brain) (9–11).

Figure 8.1 shows a Medtronic DBS device, which displays the DBS lead that is inserted into the brain, connector wire, and neurostimulator (battery).

How does the neurosurgeon get the DBS lead to the exact spot in my brain that will help my PD?

The entire DBS procedure is designed to be as minimally invasive as possible. The technology has advanced to such an extent that high-quality brain scans combined with advanced mathematics can (in a field referred to as stereotactic surgery) achieve millimeter-size precision to facilitate hitting multiple possible brain targets.

The way a typical DBS operation proceeds is as follows. First, a patient undergoes an MRI scan the day prior to surgery (takes about an hour) (Fig. 8.2). Then, on the day of surgery, the neurosurgeon attaches a heavy hat on the patient (referred to as a head frame). The patient then undergoes a CT scan (takes a few minutes), and while being wheeled to the operating room a computer fuses the MRI and the CT scan together (Fig. 8.3). The low-quality CT scan is replaced with the high-quality MRI. The markers on the

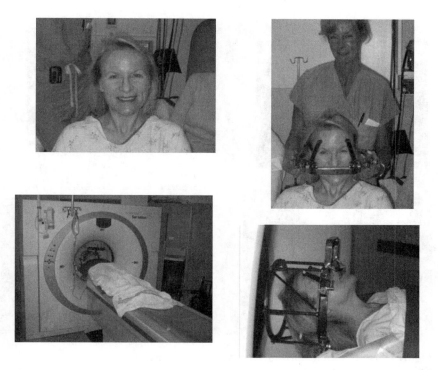

Figure 8.2 A patient before DBS (top left). Application of the head frame (top right). The patient during a computed tomography scan (bottom left). The patient with the head frame and a device with markers attached to the head frame that will assist in CT-MRI fusion for more accurate targeting (bottom right).

head frame (derived from the CT scan) are maintained and these allow the brain space to be turned into what is referred to as a Cartesian coordinate system. By using reference markers in the brain, targeting is accomplished in a virtual reality space. The neurosurgeon then drills a dime-sized hole and follows a safe trajectory when placing small recording leads (micro-electrodes) or the final lead. The chosen path is purposely planned to be far away from blood vessels or other dangerous brain areas. Microelectrode recording and macrostimulation (test stimulation through the final lead) can then be used to refine the position of the final electrode (Fig. 8.4) (6).

What is microelectrode recording and why is it important?

The success of a DBS procedure is largely dependent on placing the DBS lead within millimeters of its intended target (12). To accomplish this task, neurologists, neurosurgeons, and neurophysiologists have employed

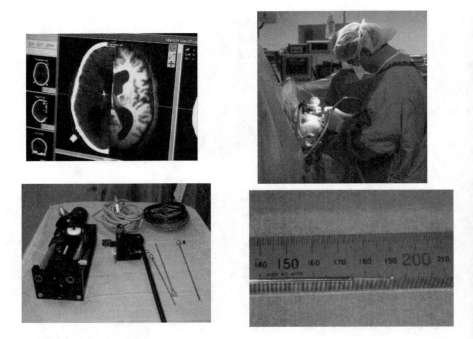

Figure 8.3 A CT (left portion) and MRI (right portion) fusion study (top left). The low-quality CT will be replaced with a high-quality MRI scan for more accurate targeting. A neurosurgeon drilling a burr hole (top right). A microelectrode recording apparatus (bottom left) and a microelectrode (bottom right).

a technology called a microelectrode. The tip of the microelectrode is approximately the size of a hair (measured in microns), and it allows the doctors to sneak up on single brain cells and eavesdrop on them. Each of the cells will sing a song (heard through headphones by a neurologist or neurophysiologist in the operating room) and based on that song a map can be drawn of their specific locations. In addition, within the operating room the doctors can passively move the face, arm, and leg and look for cells that respond to the movement, or alternatively they can stimulate the microelectrode to evoke changes in the visual or motor system. All of the information gleaned during microelectrode recording is used to form a neuroanatomical map to improve the final DBS lead placement (4,6).

Once the microelectrode mapping has been completed the surgeon will place the DBS lead. Before permanently securing the device it can be turned to an on position to confirm that the side effect to benefit threshold is reasonable for final placement (this is referred to as macrostimulation) (13–14).

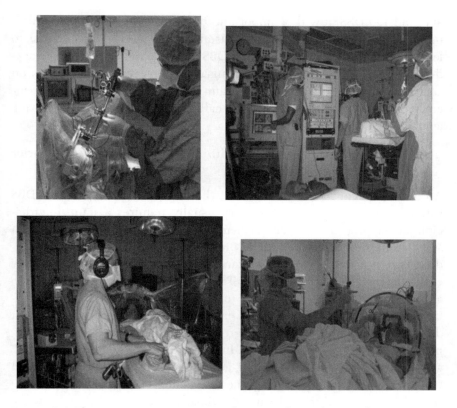

Figure 8.4 The neurosurgeon inserting the microelectrode recording apparatus into the brain (top left). A neurologist and fellow in training reading the oscilloscope, which visually reveals the brain signal (top right). A neurologist moving the leg and listening for changes in brain neuronal firing patterns (bottom left). A neurologist testing the patient (macrostimulation) once the DBS lead has been placed (bottom right).

Not all groups use microelectrode recording (15–16); however, since location is such a crucial factor in outcome, most experts highly recommend its use, and that it be used by a trained and experienced team.

What are the various disorders DBS may be performed in, and how many PWPs may be eligible?

DBS of specific targets in the brain has become an increasingly popular approach for the treatment of PD, essential tremor, dystonia, and other neurological and neuropsychiatric disorders. DBS is not for every PD, and it is estimated that only 10% to 20% of PWPs may have a favorable risk to benefit ratio with current technology. As more patients are identified and undergo DBS, it will be important for clinicians (general physicians, neurologists, nurses, physician's assistants, and nurse practitioners) to learn to recognize ideal candidates. DBS is now moving beyond the academic research centers, and its expansion has placed new demands on community practitioners. The community-based neurologist and the general practitioner will be increasingly called upon to assist with selecting appropriate DBS candidates (6,7,10).

What does it mean to have a multi/interdisciplinary screening prior to DBS, and why is it important?

An important concept to understand when evaluating any potential DBS candidate is that successful surgery usually requires a multi/interdisciplinary approach. The general neurologist or general practitioner can serve an important role in identifying and in triaging potential DBS candidates. Once triaged, potential candidates should be comprehensively evaluated by an experienced team. These teams should optimally include a movement disorders neurologist (or a neurologist experienced in evaluating movement disorders, and a neurologist experienced in movement disorders scale administration, a stereotactic-trained neurosurgeon, a neuropsychologist, a psychiatrist, and in some cases physical, occupational, and speech therapists). In addition, adequate imaging must be performed (usually an MRI and/or CT), and the results of each part of the screening should be discussed in a DBS meeting/board. These meetings/boards are usually similar in format to medical oncology boards, which are charged with deciding on the best comprehensive tumor therapy approach for both the patient and the family. The group should meet, exchange findings, and then stratify the risk benefit ratio for each patient. The multi/interdisciplinary group should be aware of and address the list of symptoms that a patient "expects" will improve with surgery. The results of this team meeting should be shared with the patient and the family to be sure that these expectations may be reasonably addressed by the recommended approach to therapy (6,17,18).

Who is a good candidate for DBS?

Probably the most crucial step for successful DBS is careful patient selection. Careful consideration of patient characteristics will directly influence outcome. Despite the widespread use of DBS, there are no standardized criteria for selection of candidates. Generally, the most suitable candidates have few other medical ailments, few if any, cognitive deficits, and a stable psychiatric status. The ideal candidate for PD surgery has fluctuating symptoms with medication-related side effects and complications of therapy (wearing off, motor fluctuations, and/or dyskinesia). DBS is a powerful treatment for smoothing out on-off fluctuations and for treating dyskinesia. Potential candidates should always be screened by experienced multi/interdisciplinary teams (6,17,18–19).

If I sign up for DBS what kind of commitment is required?

DBS requires a significant time commitment, and patients and families must be motivated to undergo not only the procedure but also the challenges associated with the preoperative work-up and the significant follow-up after the procedure. The family must be willing to return for multiple evaluations and realize that the average patient is programmed 4 to 8 times in the first 6 months following surgery. Most experienced centers have begun to shy away from performing DBS in patients unless there is a spouse or a committed caregiver (especially a caregiver that can provide travel). Many patients and families are under the erroneous impression that DBS therapy is a "light switch," and once they are turned on, the journey comes to an abrupt and miraculous end. The truth is that following activation of the device there are still many battles to be endured with both DBS programming (there are thousands of potential settings) and medication changes. Patients and families must be willing to agree to multiple programming and to medication adjustments. Patients can ultimately become DBS failures simply from a lack of commitment to the process (12).

Is DBS a cure?

There have been many television stories and news reports documenting the vivid images of lives miraculously changed by DBS. It is not hard to imagine how many people would translate the pre- and postoperative pictures to mean that DBS "cures." The reality is that although DBS is a powerful symptomatic treatment for many for the motor symptoms of PD, it is not a cure for this chronic progressive disorder. DBS will usually continue to work over many years but only for the symptoms that "continue" to be responsive to the administration of dopaminergic medications. Once symptoms such as walking, talking, and thinking become medication resistant, DBS will no longer be effective (17).

How come my doctor failed to inform me DBS would not improve my thinking (cognitive) ability?

Patient expectations must be realistic and should be discussed early in the surgical evaluation process. False expectations may represent common reasons for "DBS failures." It is sometimes useful to write out your expectations and hand them to the doctor requesting they be discussed and then documented in a chart note. If expectations shift postoperatively, you can return to the previous notes, refresh, and refocus the discussion. Open communication will keep everyone (doctors, patient, and family) in a reasonable state of mind while trying to manage inevitable device and medication issues (12,17).

What symptoms of my PD profile will respond to DBS?

In PD, the symptoms that improve with levodopa (dopamine) are generally the individual symptoms that will improve with surgery. There are a few potential exceptions to the "rule of levodopa responsiveness" including medication refractory tremor and medication refractory dyskinesia (6). Some of the most common misconceptions encountered are unrealistic patient expectations with regard to anticipated improvements in postural instability, gait, balance, and freezing. These problems in the PWP usually do not improve following DBS, unless proven to be preoperatively medication responsive with an on-off levodopa test. Patients should be cautioned that medications may or may not be reduced following DBS and that medication reduction is not the ultimate goal of the intervention. We find the following mnemonic device useful for patient education useful (17).

DBS in PD

DBS is not a cure.
Bilateral DBS is often required to improve gait.
Improves tremor, rigidity, bradykinesia, and dyskinesia
Never improves symptoms that are unresponsive to levodopa
Programming and medication adjustment are required.
Decreases medications in many, but not in all cases.

A good rule to remember is that symptoms improving with preoperative levodopa will usually improve with DBS. The UPDRS on-off levodopa motor scale is a simple bedside test that can be performed and the improvement(s) can be used to evaluate the symptoms that may respond following the operation (18).

If I have a levodopa-unresponsive parkinsonian syndrome (eg, MSA or PSP), will my symptoms respond to DBS?

When deciding on PD surgery, accurate diagnosis of what type of PD you have is a crucial determination. Patients with Parkinson plus or parkinsonian syndromes (multiple system atrophy, progressive supranuclear palsy, corticobasal degeneration, Lewy body disease, vascular parkinsonism, etc.) are not considered as candidates at this time for the current DBS technology. These other diagnoses should be excluded in the DBS screening process (6,12). Perhaps in the future new targets and technologies may make DBS available for these alternative diagnoses.

How is the on-off dopaminergic evaluation (UPDRS) obtained?

The on-off dopaminergic evaluation is a critical component to evaluating the candidacy for DBS. We prefer to evaluate the patient 12 hours "off" dopaminergic medication, using the motor section of the UPDRS—part III (this scale and a training tape for administration of the scale is available from the Movement Disorders Society). We routinely administer a suprathreshold dosage (one and a half times the regular dose) of levodopa (dopamine and all dopaminergics including dopamine agonists) to assess for levodopa responsive symptoms. The symptoms that improve with medication usually predict the ones that will improve following DBS. The on-off evaluation will also provide a useful educational tool and an excellent reminder for discussion of preoperative DBS expectations. A majority of DBS candidates usually have a minimum improvement of 30% in the UPDRS when comparing off versus on states, but there are exceptions (such as medication refractory tremor and severe dyskinesia) (18,20).

How many years should I have PD symptoms before I consider surgery?

An important consideration when contemplating DBS surgery is the duration of parkinsonian symptoms. It is preferable to consider patients candidates only if they have had symptoms for five or more years. Waiting five years will help to weed out cases of other parkinsonian syndromes. These "other" syndromes in some cases initially appear levodopa or dopamine responsive, but over 5 years in many cases they will trend toward levodopa unresponsiveness. There are exceptions to the 5-year rule, even in cases of pure PD. For example, patients with severe symptoms such as on-off fluctuations, dyskinesias, and medication refractory tremor may be operated in exceptional cases prior to a 5-year disease duration (6).

There are now several research trials examining whether there are advantages to offering DBS surgery earlier in the course of PD (6).

Will my age and other medical conditions affect my DBS candidacy?

There is no formal age limitation for DBS surgery, although the general "expert" experience has revealed that younger patients seem to experience fewer complications (6,18). There have been recent conflicting studies on whether age affects outcome in DBS. A recent study revealed that PWPs younger than 69 years suffered fewer cognitive complications. Many DBS teams feel that postoperative confusion and cognitive difficulties occur less frequently in younger patients. As potential surgical candidates age, their brains become smaller (referred to as brain atrophy), and at a certain threshold point this may increase their propensity for bleeding. Each patient must therefore be completely evaluated in all aspects of their surgical candidacy and should not be simply eliminated because they are above an arbitrary age threshold (19,21,22).

Other illnesses you may have should be carefully addressed prior to consideration of DBS surgery. Cardiac, pulmonary, and other comorbid conditions may increase the surgical risk. Obesity also will increase the surgical risk. Subjects with diabetes or those subjects who have the propensity for poor wound healing may present with increased infection risks (6,18).

Patients with hypertension have a higher risk of bleeding with micro-electrode recording (23), and therefore hypertension should be treated aggressively preoperatively and during the DBS operation.

Finally, patients must be awake during DBS surgery (in most circumstances) and participate in the procedure by providing feedback to the neurologist and neurosurgeon; therefore a healthy and cooperative subject is important for success.

Should I have a unilateral or bilateral procedure (one lead on one side of my brain or a lead placed on each side of my brain)?

Procedures may be performed unilaterally and staged (one side at a time), or bilaterally and simultaneously. It is unknown whether unilateral or staged bilateral procedures are safer. But many experts believe that there may be less adverse events when using either unilateral surgery or unilateral staged surgery (24–26). There are symptoms such as unilateral tremor that may be more amenable to a single lead placement, while gait problems or dyskinesia on both sides of the body may require bilateral implantations (18).

There are several ongoing trials examining unilateral and bilateral DBS including the NINDS/VA DBS versus Best Medical Therapy (BMT) trial, VA Effects of DBS for the Treatment of PD, the University of Amsterdam's Bilateral Internal Pallidum Stimulation in Primary Generalized Dystonia, and NINDS/VA DBS for Treatment of PD.

Our best recommendation is to choose a treatment based on a tailored and highly individualized process so that safety and efficacy can be maximized.

Why do I need neurocognitive (thinking) testing prior to and potentially following DBS?

Assessment for cognitive dysfunction is a critical portion of the presurgical evaluation. Formal neuropsychological evaluation is recommended for all patients considering DBS. When testing reveals deficits in neuropsychological testing, especially in frontal lobe and memory domains, some patients may not be suitable candidates and may be at risk for worsening with DBS surgery.

Medications can confound (worsen and cloud the picture) the performance on neuropsychological measures, so testers should be cognizant of both the disease states and the potential effects of medications taken before and during the testing. Common mistakes include testing on benzodiazepines (eg, valium and clonazepam) and pain medications and anticholinergics (cogentin, trihexyphenidyl, artane, ethopropazine, etc.) that may cloud the picture and lead to an erroneous impression a patient is demented. Another infrequent, but also potentially worrisome, scenario is the PWP whose cognition declines when their dopaminergics wear off (sometimes during testing). We believe it is essential that all patients regardless of diagnosis should undergo neuropsychological screening (18,19).

There are many brain targets that the DBS lead may be placed within. Which one should I choose?

There are three brain targets that have been FDA approved for use in PD. The most commonly used brain targets include the subthalamic nucleus (STN) and the globus pallidus interna (GPi). Target choice should be tailored to a patient's individual needs (4,9,10,18). There are many ongoing studies that will help us to refine target choice for individual patients. Although the picture is not yet clear on the issue of target choice, the STN does seem to provide more medication reduction, while GPi may be slightly safer for language and cognition. The thalamic target (VIM) is a powerful tremor suppressor, but because it has less effectiveness against the other symptoms of PD (stiffness, slowness, on-off fluctuations), either STN or GPi are used instead of VIM most of the time (4,17,18,27).

Figures 8.5–8.7 illustrate each of the three main DBS targets used in PD.

What are the complications of DBS?

DBS has many short- and long-term "potential" complications. Despite the complications that may be encountered, the vast majority of patients rate

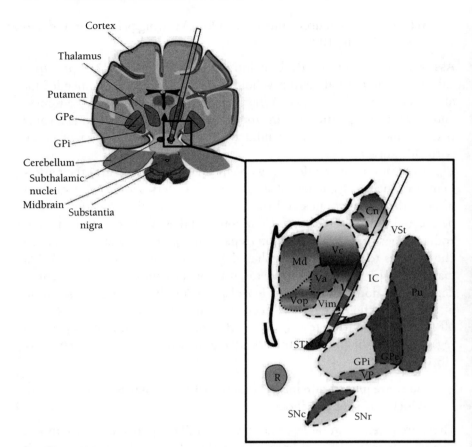

Figure 8.5 Brain target for placement of the lead in deep brain stimulation: subthalamic nucleus. Cn, caudate nucleus; GPe, globus pallidus extema; GPi, globus pallidus intema; IC, internal capsule; Md, nucleus medio dorsal thalamus; Pu, putamen; R, red nucleus; SNc, substantia nigra pars reticulate; Va, nucleus ventral anterior thalamus; Vc, nucleus ventro caudal thalamus; Vim, nucleus ventral intermedius thalamus; Vop, nucleus ventral oral posterios thalamus; VP, visual pathway/optic tract; VSt, ventral striatum; Zi, zona inserta. (Courtesy of Michael S. Okun, MD).

their experience with DBS as overwhelmingly positive. The DBS device does not have a blood supply, so infection is a primary worry and can occur in 5% or more of implanted devices. One of the biggest worries is that the microelectrodes and/or the DBS lead will injure a blood vessel resulting in bleeding, or alternatively in a stroke that may lead to weakness, numbness, changes in vision, and/or changes in speech. The DBS device can fracture/

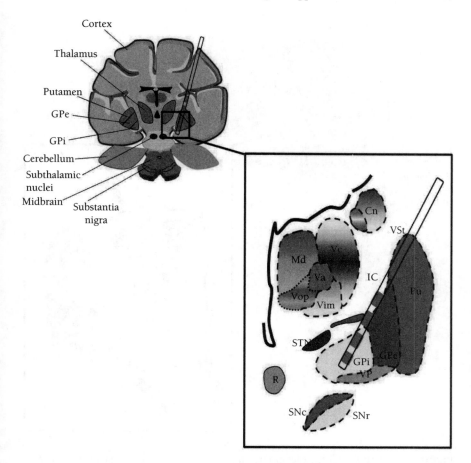

Figure 8.6 Brain target for placement of the lead in deep brain stimulation: globus pallidus intema. Cn, caudate nucleus; GPe, globus pallidus extema; GPi, globus pallidus intema; IC, internal capsule; Md, nucleus medio dorsal thalamus; Pu, putamen; R, red nucleus; SNc, substantia nigra pars reticulate; Va, nucleus ventral anterior thalamus; Vc, nucleus ventro caudal thalamus; Vim, nucleus ventral intermedius thalamus; Vop, nucleus ventral oral posterios thalamus; VP, visual pathway/optic tract; VSt, ventral striatum; Zi, zona inserta. (Courtesy of Michael S. Okun, MD).

break, migrate out of position, or malfunction. In addition, only levodopa-responsive symptoms can be expected to improve; therefore, with disease progression, walking, talking, and thinking may all evolve to become part of the disease syndrome. DBS commonly affects the speech, and particularly verbal fluency (getting words out of the mouth). There can be worsening of cognition or mood, and in rare cases associated suicidal thoughts

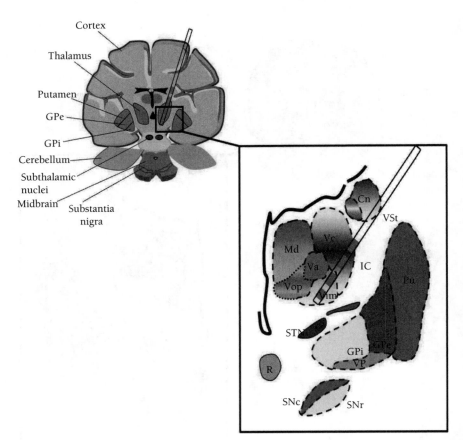

Figure 8.7 Brain target for placement of the lead in deep brain stimulation: ventral intermediate nucleus. Cn, caudate nucleus; GPe, globus pallidus extema; GPi, globus pallidus intema; IC, internal capsule; Md, nucleus medio dorsal thalamus; Pu, putamen; R, red nucleus; SNc, substantia nigra pars reticulate; Va, nucleus ventral anterior thalamus; Vc, nucleus ventro caudal thalamus; Vim, nucleus ventral intermedius thalamus; Vop, nucleus ventral oral posterios thalamus; VP, visual pathway/optic tract; VSt, ventral striatum; Zi, zona inserta. (Courtesy of Michael S. Okun, MD).

(another reason why patients must be carefully screened and followed). The addition of a second DBS lead in the opposite brain may also increase the risk for walking, talking, and thinking problems (16,28,29).

The biggest risk of a DBS procedure is failure to achieve the patient's preoperative expectations, and this is why it is critical that both patients and physicians have focused preoperative discussions (12,17,18).

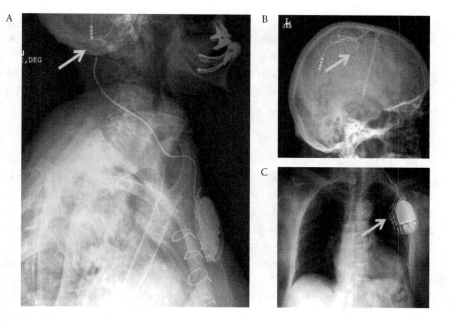

Figure 8.8 An X-ray of a patient showing placement of the DBS lead and device. (A) There is discontinuity in the deep brain stimulator wiring at the level of the left mastoid process (ear) from the battery pack and also (B,C) the electrode is coiled in the extracranial soft tissues.

Figure 8.6 shows a plain x-ray film series through the skull, neck, and chest of a DBS patient with a deep brain stimulator coursing through the neck and terminating in the left chest wall.

I feel electric shock–like sensations in my head and neck. What is that?

When the DBS hardware is damaged, an electrical short may develop. The clinical manifestation of a short may be an electric sensation. Sometimes this sensation manifests when the hardware or wire under the skin is palpated. If this occurs, you should visit your doctor immediately. The DBS programmer in your doctor's office can check the wires to evaluate for electrical shorts, and also for fractures. In addition, your doctor in some cases may need to send you for plain film x-rays to try to identify the area of the damage so that it can be repaired or replaced (12,19).

I have heard there can be DBS failures. What does that mean?

A DBS failure occurs when a patient has a DBS device implanted and is unsatisfied for any number of reasons regarding benefit and/or side effects. A recent publication on this topic cites that most DBS failures are preventable when a multi/interdisciplinary DBS team is used and when there are adequate triage, screening, performance of the procedure, programming, and medication adjustments. A breakdown in any of these areas or the lack of availability DBS management services may lead to a DBS failure (12,19).

What do I do if I am having problems with my DBS device?

If you are having problems with your DBS device, it is best to see an experienced DBS team. A recent publication has outlined procedures to deal with troubleshooting DBS devices (19). The first step is for your doctor to take a detailed patient history. Then, we recommend that the UPDRS standardized PD scale be obtained in the off-medication–on-DBS condition, the off medication off DBS condition, the on medication off DBS condition, and the on medication on DBS condition. The responses in each of these conditions should offer a clue as to whether the DBS is functioning as well as expected (using the performance scores versus the medications). Next, the device should be carefully imaged, and then a programmer should record thresholds for side effects and benefits at each contact and attempt reprogramming as well as medication adjustment. The DBS multi/interdisciplinary team can then review all of these findings and decide on the best management strategies, which may or may not be reoperation (30). We have found in many cases that reoperation can be beneficial for select patients.

I have speech problems when my DBS is on. Can it be reprogrammed?

Speech problems are among the most common side effects encountered with DBS (31–33). The device can be reprogrammed from monopolar (wide field strength) to bipolar (narrow field strength) in some cases, and this may result in improvement in symptoms. Also, some patients may switch off their devices with a remote control in situations where they need to speak but may have less of a need for control of motor symptoms (eg, tremor and stiffness). In general, the treatment of speech problems resulting from DBS has been challenging. We sometimes employ LSVTs as well as speech and swallowing consultations, but in many cases we are unable to obtain a satisfactory benefit for patients despite all approaches. It is important to be aware preoperatively that speech volume and verbal fluency may be adversely affected by DBS and that your doctors may not be able to reprogram the device or employ rehabilitative strategies to overcome the deficits. There is some evidence that the verbal fluency problems in STN DBS may in some cases persist even in the DBS off state.

All of my PD symptoms are under control except my gait and balance. Should I have DBS?

STN and/or GPi DBS should only be employed for levodopa responsive gait, balance, and freezing problems. DBS cannot be expected to improve these symptoms if they are not responding to medications, and you should be aware that as PD progresses you might encounter these symptoms with or without DBS (18).

There is some new promising research that targets a levodopa-resistant gait and balance issues (34); but more research needs to be done to evaluate which patients will be the best candidates for this new DBS brain target.

Are there any laws governing who can program DBS?

That is an excellent question, and although we do not know the legal answer, we highly encourage people to have the device programmed only by a trained expert and not by a company representative. In our practice only the physicians, nurses, and physicians in training are allowed to program devices and examine patients. We do not endorse the idea of random and untrained people changing DBS settings, as we have learned that there is a delicate balance to be struck for success—and also there can be issues that arise acutely and chronically from individual programming settings. These issues may require emergency visits, medication changes, the use of a multi/interdisciplinary team, and/or DBS adjustment in settings.

Since having my DBS my medications have not changed. When I am medicated I am fine, with no problems. Should I have more electric stimulation or less? Or should rate and pulse width be changed?

This question is impossible to answer precisely without seeing and examining you; however, there are a few generalities that may be helpful in guiding you to the answer. DBSs for PD are implanted and then we usually employ a 30-day waiting period for brain swelling to subside. Then, following resolution of brain swelling, we adjust the DBS and the medications about once a month for six months. Although our goal is not medication reduction, in many cases medications can be changed and this may include dose, number of medications, and medication interval. We adjust the DBS device by having patients attend a DBS specialty clinic "off" of their medications overnight. Following the session, we may recommend medication adjustments, and we generally make these adjustments slowly over many months (it takes months to adjust the balance between medications and DBS). Unilateral DBS usually allows for less reduction in medications than bilateral DBS, and it is felt that certain targets may be more amenable to medication reduction (eg, STN). Usually 6 months postsurgery, the DBS settings are close to or completely optimized, and from that point forward the mainstay of therapy is medication change with only slight changes in DBS settings (voltage, pulse width, frequency). We have to be careful to discourage patients from requesting frequent changes after optimization has been achieved, as DBS will only improve symptoms equivalent to the best medication on state and further tinkering has the potential to worsen their clinical states.

Is DBS available in all countries?

DBS is just one example of a therapy that when offered to well-selected patients has the potential to dramatically change their lives. There are many more examples of this in PD including medical, surgical, and behavioral therapies. It is important that we launch initiatives through NPF and other organizations to address the world's needs for these new therapies. Dr. Fernandez recently launched a program in Philippines called SUPPORT-PD this year, and all of the "ask the doctors" from our forums participated (Drs Rodriguez, Foote, Okun). We worked with the Filipino doctors for 1 year helping them set up a referral network and an interdisciplinary surgical team. We then lectured for a week in their country, increased awareness, built enthusiasm, and assisted in two DBS surgeries. They have now developed a terrific multi/interdisciplinary DBS program. We need to continue to expand education and outreach all over the planet to be sure that people who can benefit from DBS will benefit.

Why shouldn't I just have gamma knife radiosurgery for PD?

Gamma knife or radiosurgery for PD is an alternative that has been widely publicized in recent years. One advantage to radiosurgery is that the procedure can be done without an incision (simply using radiation pointed at the brain target to accomplish the lesion). However, there are many disadvantages in this type of surgery, particularly when compared to standard DBS. In radiosurgery, the benefits are delayed and interestingly the side effects may also be delayed (showing up weeks to months later). The gamma knife lesion is a destructive one and therefore irreversible and is of inferior accuracy compared to what can be obtained by DBS. If the radiation lesions "run away," unintended structures may become involved in the lesion and side effects may occur. Finally, unlike DBS, gamma knife radiosurgery cannot be programmed or adjusted. Radiosurgery, however, may be an option for a small number of patients who have a high risk for surgical complications if a standard DBS procedure is elected—such as those on blood thinners, or who have other major medical issues (35).

REFERENCES

1. Benabid AL, Koudsié A, Benazzouz A, et al. Subthalamic stimulation for Parkinson's disease. *Arch Med Res.* 2000;31(3):282–289.
2. Benabid AL, Krack PP, Benezzouz A, Limousin P, Koudsie A, Pollak P. Deep brain stimulation of the subthalamic nucleus for Parkinson's disease: methodologic aspects and clinical criteria. *Neurology.* 2000;55(12 suppl 6):S40–S44.
3. Okun MS, Foote KD. A mnemonic for Parkinson disease patients considering DBS: a tool to improve perceived outcome of surgery. *Neurologist.* 2004;10(5):290.
4. Okun MS, Vitek JL. Lesion therapy for Parkinson's disease and other movement disorders: update and controversies. *Mov Disord.* 2004;19(4):375–389.
5. Okun MS, Rodriguez RL, Mikos A, et al. Deep brain stimulation and the role of the neuropsychologist. *Clin Neuropsychol.* 2007;21(1):162–189.
6. Okun MS, Fernandez HH, Rodriguez RL, Foote KD. Identifying candidates for deep brain stimulation in Parkinson's disease: the role of the primary care physician. *Geriatrics.* 2007;62(5):18–24.
7. Greenberg BD, Askland KD, Carpenter LL. The evolution of deep brain stimulation for neuropsychiatric disorders. *Front Biosci.* 2008;13:4638–4648.
8. Greenberg BD, Gabriels LA, Malone DA Jr, et al. Deep brain stimulation of the ventral internal capsule/ventral striatum for obsessive-compulsive disorder: worldwide experience. *Mol Psychiatry.* 2008;
9. Benabid AL, Benazzouz A, Hoffmann D, Limousin P. Long-term electrical inhibition of deep brain targets in movement disorders. *Mov Disord.* 1998;13(suppl):119–125.
10. Benabid AL, Chabardes, S, Seigneuret E. Deep-brain stimulation in Parkinson's disease: long-term efficacy and safety—what happened this year? *Curr Opin Neurol.* 2005;18(6):623–630.
11. Benabid AL. What the future holds for deep brain stimulation. *Expert Rev Med Devices.* 2007;4(6):895–903.
12. Okun MS, Tagliati M, Pourfar M, et al. Management of referred deep brain stimulation failures: a retrospective analysis from 2 movement disorders centers. *Arch Neurol.* 2005;62(8):1250–1255.
13. Vitek JL, Ashe J, DeLong MR, Kaneoke Y. Microstimulation of primate motor thalamus: somatotopic organization and differential distribution of evoked motor responses among subnuclei. *J Neurophysiol.* 1996;75(6):2486–2495.
14. Vitek JL, Bakay RA, DeLong MR. Microelectrode-guided pallidotomy for medically intractable Parkinson's disease. *Adv Neurol.* 1997;74:183–198.
15. Hariz MI, Fodstad H. Do microelectrode techniques increase accuracy or decrease risks in pallidotomy and deep brain stimulation? A critical review of the literature. *Stereotact Funct Neurosurg.* 1999;72(2–4):157–169.

16. Hariz MI. Safety and risk of microelectrode recording in surgery for movement disorders. *Stereotact Funct Neurosurg.* 2002;78(3–4):146–157.

17. Okun MS, Foote KD. Subthalamic nucleus vs globus pallidus interna deep brain stimulation, the rematch: will pallidal deep brain stimulation make a triumphant return? *Arch Neurol.* 2005;62(4):533–536.

18. Rodriguez RL, Fernandez HH, Haq I, Okun MS. Pearls in patient selection for deep brain stimulation. *Neurologist.* 2007;13(5):253–260.

19. Okun MS, Rodriguez RL, Foote KD, et al. A case-based review of troubleshooting deep brain stimulator issues in movement and neuropsychiatric disorders. *Parkinsonism Relat Disord.* 2007;14(7):532–538.

20. Charles PD, Van Blercom N, Krack P, et al. Predictors of effective bilateral subthalamic nucleus stimulation for PD. *Neurology.* 2002;59(6):932–934.

21. Pillon B, Ardouin C, Damier P, et al. Neuropsychological changes between "off" and "on" STN or GPi stimulation in Parkinson's disease. *Neurology.* 2000;55(3):411–418.

22. Saint-Cyr JA, Trépanier LL, Kumar R, Lozano AM, Lang AE. Neuropsychological consequences of chronic bilateral stimulation of the subthalamic nucleus in Parkinson's disease. *Brain.* 2000;123(pt 10):2091–2108.

23. Gorgulho A, De Salles AA, Frighetto L, Behnke E. Incidence of hemorrhage associated with electrophysiological studies performed using macroelectrodes and microelectrodes in functional neurosurgery. *J Neurosurg.* 2005;102(5):888–896.

24. Alberts JL, Elder CM, Okun MS, Vitek JL. Comparison of pallidal and subthalamic stimulation on force control in patient's with Parkinson's disease. *Motor Control.* 2004;8(4):484–499.

25. Alberts JL, Hass CJ, Okun MS, Vitek JL. Are two leads always better than one: an emerging case for unilateral subthalamic deep brain stimulation in Parkinson's disease. *Exp Neurol.* 2008;

26. Alberts JL, Okun MS, Vitek JL. The persistent effects of unilateral pallidal and subthalamic deep brain stimulation on force control in advanced Parkinson's patients. *Parkinsonism Relat Disord.* 2008;14(6):481–488.

27. Espay AJ, Duker AP, Chen R, et al. Deep brain stimulation of the ventral intermediate nucleus of the thalamus in medically refractory orthostatic tremor: preliminary observations. *Mov Disord.* 2008;23(16):2357–2362.

28. Hariz MI, Rehncrona S, Quinn NP, Speelman JD, Wensing C. Multicenter study on deep brain stimulation in Parkinson's disease: an independent assessment of reported adverse events at 4 years. *Mov Disord.* 2008;23(3):416–421.

29. Videnovic A, Metman LV. Deep brain stimulation for Parkinson's disease: prevalence of adverse events and need for standardized reporting. *Mov Disord.* 2008;23(3):343–349.

30. Ellis TM, Foote KD, Fernandez HH, et al. Reoperation for suboptimal outcomes after deep brain stimulation surgery. *Neurosurgery.* 2008;63(4):754–760; discussion 760–761.

31. Krack P, Batir A, Van Blercom N, et al. Five-year follow-up of bilateral stimulation of the subthalamic nucleus in advanced Parkinson's disease. *N Engl J Med.* 2003;349(20):1925–1934.

32. Bruce BB, Foote KD, Rosenbeck J, et al. Aphasia and thalamotomy: important issues. *Stereotact Funct Neurosurg.* 2004;82(4):186–190.

33. Benabid AL, Chabardes S, Seigneuret E. Functional neurosurgery: past, present, and future. *Clin Neurosurg.* 2005;(52):265–270.

34. Kenney C, Fernandez HH, Okun MS. Role of deep brain stimulation targeted to the pedunculopontine nucleus in Parkinson's disease. *Expert Rev Neurother.* 2007;7(6):585–589.

35. Okun MS, Stover NP, Subramanian T, et al. Complications of gamma knife surgery for Parkinson disease. *Arch Neurol.* 2001;58(12):1995–2002.

In China they are performing stem cell surgery for Parkinson's disease. I'm considering going to China to have the surgery done. I am 63 years old, happily married, diagnosed 3 years ago but my symptoms probably started 5 years ago. I am still able to walk, talk, and enjoy myself for the most part, but I want this disease out of my system! I would appreciate any comments negative or positive from you on this procedure.

CHAPTER 9

Stem Cells, Gene Therapy, Transplants, and Other Medical Treatments

What is a stem cell?

Stem cells are immature cells in the body that can differentiate into one of many body tissues (1).

One analogy of the power of a stem cell would be to compare it to a child. Early in development, parents can influence a child to differentiate into one or another area of life and to develop a skill set for success in adulthood. Stem cells are a potentially self-renewing resource that can be influenced by scientists to differentiate (change) into a needed tissue (1–3).

Previously, most research efforts were geared toward the harvesting (obtaining) of stem cells from discarded human embryos (4,5). This type of stem cell harvesting has drawn the most controversy, mainly from religious groups with deep-seated beliefs that obtaining the cells in this manner is both unethical and against the practices of the church. Recently, however, neurogenesis has been proven to occur in the adult human brain (1,6,7). Neurogenesis, or the formation of new cells from existing adult human brain tissue, has been an important discovery in the past decade of stem cell research. There is a region of the brain called the subventricular zone (a zone very close to the water carrying areas of the brain called the ventricles), which is known to be rich in stem cells and has been referred to as brain marrow (with the comparison to bone marrow, where blood stem cells reside) (1). There are now major research efforts directed toward

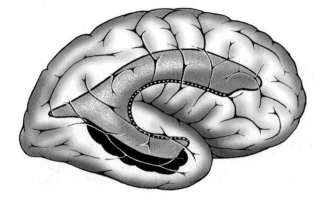

Figure 9.1 The subventricular zone in the brain. The darker gray area in the center of the diagram represents the water carrying area of the brain (the cerebrospinal fluid), and the white dots on the black background represent the stem cells. (Courtesy of Dennis A. Steindler, PhD).

the development of these adult stem cells that have now also been identified in other regions of the brain including the hippocampus (1–3,6–9).

Figure 9.1 is a diagram of the brain showing where the subventricular stem cells live.

What are the problems/challenges of stem cells for PD?

There are significant problems with stem cells as a potential savior therapy for PD. First, when you take a cell and make it divide you must be able to turn it on and off. If you cannot control growth of the cells, then they have the potential to form cancers. This limitation of stem cell therapy is an area that has drawn increasing attention from researchers and funding organizations, and pairing stem cell therapy with gene therapy, for example, may help to alleviate this issue. The other major issue with stem cell therapy is that it fails to address the complexity of PD. PD was long thought to be a simple loss of dopaminergic cells part of the brain. We are now aware that there is a much greater level of complexity to this disease and that multiple motor and nonmotor circuits and regions (10,11) throughout the brain area were affected. In addition, PD may actually be combination of multiple diseases with similar manifestations. These issues may prove limiting for stem cells or for any transplantation strategy. An important area of research, therefore, will need to be investigation into "how to encourage stem cells" to repopulate and repair multiple brain circuits in many brain regions (1–3,5,6,9,12,13).

How will stem cell research be affected by changes in the political administration?

It is a complex issue. One very positive sign is that the Obama administration has signaled a willingness to reopen the area of the development
of embryonic stem cell lines for use in PD and other neurodegenerative
diseases. This move will immediately free stem cell scientists previously
limited to a number of existing stem cell lines that were capped by the
current administration. Though this move will not directly affect the adult
stem cell researchers, the indirect impact may be significant. Adult stem
cell researchers have been hampered by a general sense of political nega-
tivity about the use of any stem cell for the treatment or cure of a neurological disease. In addition, they have been handcuffed by state governments
and funding agencies caught in the political question of embryonic stem
cell research, even though their approaches should be noncontroversial.
Therefore, there is hope that with government support there will be a new
spirit that will trickle down to assist both embryonic and adult stem cell
researchers.

What is the potential timeline for stem cell breakthroughs in PD?

The timeline for major breakthroughs in stem cell research is at best
"fuzzy." We have been encouraged by the thoughtfulness of the scientists
involved in the research, and we remain hopeful that more breakthroughs
will emerge both with time and with the increased support of the incom-
ing presidential administration. We hope that state agencies as well as
other funding agencies will become more open to the funding of stem
cell–related projects—whether they are embryonic or adult focused. It
is important for people interested in stem cell therapies to keep in mind
that the answer may not be simply stem cell monotherapy (eg, stem cells
alone). In addition to developing on-off technology and the ability to
integrate into the brain's complex circuitry, scientists should continue to
keep open the possibility that a combination therapy (gene therapy, oral
agents, etc.) may provide a more comprehensive approach to a very complex problem.

What is gene therapy?

A common question asked by many patients and families afflicted with PD
is, "what is gene therapy?" Quite simply, gene therapy is placing genetic
information (DNA) into the cells and tissues of humans with PD (14–16).
In the purest form, a defective part of the genome is replaced with a new
copy. Perhaps the most interesting part of the evolving story of gene therapy

has been the use of a virus as a vector to carry the genetic information into the brain. These viruses have been deactivated and can be safely used for this purpose (15,17–19).

What are the current ongoing gene therapy trials for PD?

There are three large ongoing gene trials in humans with PD. The first trial aims to deliver amino acid decarboxylase (the sponsoring company is Avigen), which is a brain enzyme that may help enhance the effectiveness of dopaminergic medicines like levodopa (Sinemet), and perhaps reduce the doses drugs, and consequently their side effects (20). The second trial delivers neurturin, which is a protein that may repair and rescue dopamine cells in the brain (21). Neurturin (the sponsoring company is Ceregene) has recently been tested in a multicenter protocol (Ceregene trial), and results were disappointing. Neuturin belongs to the same protein family as glial cell–derived neurotrophic factor (GDNF), which was another gene therapy that had disappointing results in a recently publicized trial (the sponsoring company is Amgen) (22,23). The final trial focuses on an enzyme called glutamic acid decarboxylase (GAD) (the sponsoring company is Neurologix) (15,24,25).

Kaplitt and colleagues reported in *Lancet* in 2007, the "Safety and tolerability of gene therapy with an adeno-associated virus (AAV) borne GAD gene for Parkinson's disease: an open label, phase I trial" (25). The STN is a brain structure that spews a chemical called glutamate onto another structure in the brain called the globus pallidus. Many treatment schemes have focused on controlling or neuromodulating the output from the STN. One such approach has been inserting a lead into the brain and introducing electricity to change the firing pattern and rate emanating from the STN (DBS). Kaplitt and colleagues have developed the innovative approach of using gene therapy to change the STN from a chemically excitatory nucleus to a chemically inhibitory one. These investigators measured the safety, tolerability, and preliminary efficacy of the "transfer of glutamic acid decarboxylase (GAD) gene with adeno-associated virus (AAV) into the STN of patients with Parkinson's disease." The original study published in *Lancet* had 11 patients. The group was similar to those used for DBS (less than 70 with on-off motor fluctuations and minimal cognitive dysfunction). The most important outcome was "no adverse events related to the gene therapy. Significant improvements in motor UPDRS (the scale used by neurologists to measure Parkinson's disease improvement) motor scores (p=0.0015), predominantly on the side of the body that was contralateral to surgery, were seen 3 months after gene therapy and persisted up to 12 months."

The relative magnitude of the changes in the UPDRS scales seemed to be roughly similar to what has been observed following DBS, although longer term follow-up of motor symptoms will be needed. Many experts have held that gene therapy has a high "bar" to pass, as the results of DBS have provided excellent benefits in a similar group of patients. Preliminary analyses point to the benefit (similar to DBS) as being predominantly in motor function and not in areas of nonmotor or levodopa resistant symptoms (depression, sleep, gait, communication, etc.). No one knows if changing the excitatory function of the nucleus into inhibitory will affect learning, but this is a point that will require close follow-up. Perhaps the most important finding was that gene therapy was successfully used in humans with PD and that this success may open the door to future gene therapies, as well as to combination therapies (genes plus stem cells or genes plus medications, or genes plus DBS).

What is GDNF?

GDNF stands for glial cell lined–derived neurotrophic factor. GDNF is a protein that is encoded by the GDNF gene, and it functions as a fertilizer in promoting survival of brain cells. GDNF has been shown in experiments to be particularly good at promoting survival of dopamine neurons, and this is one reason so much work has been focused on it as a potential treatment in PD. Over the past decade, there has been a flurry of research laboratory activity regarding GDNF experiments in PD. Human trials to date, however, have been disappointing with the most recent trial by Amgen stopped due to lack of efficacy as well as patient safety issues. Recently, however, there has been a renewed interested in GDNF as a therapy for PD, and many scientists have suggested that lessons learned from the GDNF failures may be leveraged into future successes (26–34). In addition, other factors such as conserved dopamine neurotropic factor (CDNF) and neurturin have recently entered the field as other therapeutic possibilities.

What have been the results of transplant trials for PD?

Several preliminary open-label pilot studies of various transplant techniques for human PD were observed to have varying degrees of success. Transplants with adrenal medullary cells and then human embryonic dopaminergic cells were sought as a potential treatment for advanced PD. Two independent double-blinded studies (investigator blind and examiner blind) failed to reveal adequate efficacy when compared to a sham group (a group who received burr holes in the head but no transplant), although the younger patients seemed to display some positive motor benefits.

There are many potential reasons for the failure of the transplant trial experiences. Perhaps the most compelling reason for failure is the complex nature of the multiple motor and nonmotor circuits affected (10,11,35–37) in PD. The transplants only attempted to replace dopaminergic cells in one degenerated area of the brain (the putamen). Future approaches may need to broaden their scope to account for the many brain systems involved in PD.

The use of sham surgery or drilling burr holes in the skull but not implanting cells in half the patients in the transplant trials has drawn much ethical discussions. It is interesting that the open-label unblinded effects of the pilot surgery that led to the larger blinded trials were so positive, but when a sham group was used, the placebo effects cancelled out many of the potential benefits. In addition, the group that received the transplanted cells also developed unacceptable side effects (eg, dyskinesias), as compared to those in the sham group. Finally, if the study was positive and safe, the sham group would have been ultimately offered the transplanted cells (13,38–47).

Is it true that PWP transplants develop strange and uncontrollable dyskinesias?

Patients enrolled in both of the large double-blind placebo-controlled trials for transplantation of embryonic dopaminergic cells developed a unique and never before observed side effect referred to as runaway dyskinesia. The term runaway dyskinesia has been coined because the extra movements (or dyskinesias) occurred in both the "off" medication state as well as in the "on" medication state. Normally, dyskinesias in patients without transplants only occur in the "on" medication state. It is still speculative as to why this side effect occurred in the transplanted patients, but most experts believe that in some way the grafted tissue reconstituted the circuitry in an aberrant way (39,48,49).

Why did the imaging following the PD transplants improve, but the patients did not?

One of the most interesting findings derived from the transplant studies has been imaging data and also postmortem data that has revealed that the transplanted cells have survived and prospered in their new home. This finding is encouraging for the future of the transplant field; however, it reminds us that the gold standard for improvement is not the MRI scan, but rather the patient (48,50).

Is it true that the neurodegenerative process was found to proceed even within PD transplants?

One of the most fascinating findings that has now been reported by multiple groups is the phenomenon of spreading neurodegeneration from the host tissue into the newly grafted cells. Careful examination of postmortem brains following embryonic fetal cell transplants has shown evidence of the Lewy Body and other neurodegenerative features in the previously unaffected cells transplanted into the host. Scientists are hopeful that the explanation of this phenomenon will help unlock some of the mysteries surrounding PD (50,51).

What is Spheramine, and can it be transplanted to help PD?

Spheramine is a cell-based therapy, which was recently transplanted into the brains of PWPs in a double-blinded trial (half-got spheramine and half-got sham surgery). Spheramine consists of human retinal epithelial cells attached to what is called a microcarrier support matrix, which helps survival. One of the rationales for the study was the finding that inner retinal cells could produce dopamine. Recent positive unblinded studies led to the blinded trial, which was recently reported to have disappointing results and not meeting its primary outcome variable (47).

Should I volunteer for a PD stem cell, gene therapy, or transplant trial?

Though the preliminary results of gene therapy and transplant therapy have been mixed, we have made important progress in the field. We have achieved what is referred to as "proof of concept" in the scientific field. We have achieved some promising results, and it is likely that we will get better and better as therapies, strategies, and combination therapies and delivery systems continue to evolve. One of the reasons why PD stays ahead of many other neurological diseases is that the PWPs have shown tremendous courage and optimism in volunteering for trials and therefore in propelling therapies forward. We have learned from both our successes and our failures and, in this way, we are making it better for the next generation of therapies and for the next generation of PWPs who will receive them.

Whenever volunteering for a trial, remember to make sure that the scientific group has legitimate credentials and that the protocol has been reviewed and approved by an institutional review board to protect the interests of the participating subjects.

There are several fee-for–stem cell initiatives on the Internet with impressive data and statistics. Should I travel overseas to these programs and get a stem cell transplant?

Human stem cell transplants are not ready for prime time. We have not yet learned how to regulate stem cells (turn them on and off) and prevent them from forming tumors. In addition, the lessons learned from the embryonic transplant trials apply to stem cell transplants—mainly, it is not enough to just simply insert cells into the brain and expect them to reconstitute a complex PD circuitry. Therefore, we strongly advise against exposing yourself to the risks of a fee-for-stem cells scam, and we would encourage patients to participate only in such human transplant research that are approved and monitored by institutional review board.

REFERENCES

1. Steindler DA. Stem cells, regenerative medicine, and animal models of disease. *Ilar J.* 2007;48(4):323–338.
2. Trzaska KA, Rameshwar P. Current advances in the treatment of Parkinson's disease with stem cells. *Curr Neurovasc Res.* 2007;4(2):99–109.
3. Svendsen C. Stem cells and Parkinson's disease: toward a treatment, not a cure. *Cell Stem Cell.* 2008;2(5):412–413.
4. Brockman-Lee SA. Embryonic stem cells in science and medicine: an invitation for dialogue. *Gend Med.* 2007;4(4):288–293.
5. Xi J, Zhang SC. Stem cells in development of therapeutics for Parkinson's disease: a perspective. *J Cell Biochem.* 2008;105(5):1153–1160.
6. Arias-Carrion O, Freundlieb N, et al. Adult neurogenesis and Parkinson's disease. *CNS Neurol Disord Drug Targets.* 2007;6(5):326–335.
7. Park DH, Borlongan CV, et al. The emerging field of cell and tissue engineering. *Med Sci Monit.* 2008;14(11):RA206–RA220.
8. Andres RH, Meyer M, et al. Restorative neuroscience: concepts and perspectives. *Swiss Med Wkly.* 2008;138(11–12):155–172.
9. Deuschl G. Therapy of Parkinson's disease 2008 [in German]. *MMW Fortschr Med.* 2008;150(suppl 2):60–63.
10. Alexander GE, DeLong MR, et al. Parallel organization of functionally segregated circuits linking basal ganglia and cortex. *Annu Rev Neurosci.* 1986;9:357–381.
11. Alexander GE, Crutcher MD, et al. Basal ganglia-thalamocortical circuits: parallel substrates for motor, oculomotor, "prefrontal" and "limbic" functions. *Prog Brain Res.* 1990;85:119–146.
12. Wang Y, Chen S, et al. Stem cell transplantation: a promising therapy for Parkinson's disease. *J Neuroimmune Pharmacol.* 2007;2(3):243–250.

13. Wijeyekoon R, Barker RA. Cell replacement therapy for Parkinson's disease. *Biochim Biophys Acta.* 2008.

14. Freese A, Stern M, et al. Prospects for gene therapy in Parkinson's disease. *Mov Disord.* 1996;11(5):469–488.

15. Kaplitt MG, Pfaff DW. Viral vectors for gene delivery and expression in the CNS. *Methods.* 1996;10(3):343–350.

16. Bartus RT, Herzog CD, et al. Issues regarding gene therapy products for Parkinson's disease: the development of CERE-120 (AAV-NTN) as one reference point. *Parkinsonism Relat Disord.* 2007;13(suppl 3):S469–S477.

17. Mandel SA, Amit T, et al. Targeting multiple neurodegenerative diseases etiologies with multimodal-acting green tea catechins. *J Nutr.* 2008;138(8):1578S–1583S.

18. Palfi S. Towards gene therapy for Parkinson's disease. *Lancet Neurol.* 2008;7(5):375–376.

19. Schneider B, Zufferey R, et al. Viral vectors, animal models and new therapies for Parkinson's disease. *Parkinsonism Relat Disord.* 2008;14(suppl 2):S169–S171.

20. Eberling JL, Jagust WJ, et al. Results from a phase I safety trial of hAADC gene therapy for Parkinson disease. *Neurology.* 2008;70(21):1980–1983.

21. Marks WJ Jr, Ostrem JL, et al. Safety and tolerability of intraputaminal delivery of CERE-120 (adeno-associated virus serotype 2-neurturin) to patients with idiopathic Parkinson's disease: an open-label, phase I trial. *Lancet Neurol.* 2008;7(5):400–408.

22. Pollack A. Patients in test won't get drug, Amgen decides. New York, NY: Times (Print);2005:C1, C2.

23. Matcham JM, McDermott P, et al. GDNF in Parkinson's disease: the perils of post-hoc power. *J Neurosci Methods.* 2007;163(2):193–196.

24. During MJ, Kaplitt MG, et al. Subthalamic GAD gene transfer in Parkinson disease patients who are candidates for deep brain stimulation. *Hum Gene Ther.* 2001;12(12):1589–1591.

25. Kaplitt MG, Feigin A, et al. Safety and tolerability of gene therapy with an adeno-associated virus (AAV) borne GAD gene for Parkinson's disease: an open label, phase I trial. *Lancet.* 2007;369(9579):2097–2105.

26. Lang AE, Langston JW, et al. GDNF in treatment of Parkinson's disease: response to editorial. *Lancet Neurol.* 2006;5(3):200–202.

27. Salvatore MF, Ai Y, et al. Point source concentration of GDNF may explain failure of phase II clinical trial. *Exp Neurol.* 2006;202(2):497–505.

28. Sherer TB, Fiske BK, et al. Crossroads in GDNF therapy for Parkinson's disease. *Mov Disord.* 2006;21(2):136–141.

29. Slevin JT, Gash, DM, et al. Unilateral intraputaminal glial cell line-derived neurotrophic factor in patients with Parkinson disease: response to 1 year each of treatment and withdrawal. *Neurosurg Focus.* 2006;20(5):E1.

30. Slevin JT, Gerhardt GA, et al. Reply: GDNF poses troubling questions for doctors, drug maker. *Ann Neurol.* 2006;59(6):989–990.

31. Bespalov MM, Saarma M. GDNF family receptor complexes are emerging drug targets. *Trends Pharmacol Sci.* 2007;28(2):68–74.

32. Yasuhara T, Shingo T, et al. Glial cell line-derived neurotrophic factor (GDNF) therapy for Parkinson's disease. *Acta Med Okayama.* 2007;61(2):51–56.

33. Hong M, Mukhida K, et al. GDNF therapy for Parkinson's disease. *Expert Rev Neurother.* 2008;8(7):1125–1139.

34. Peterson AL, Nutt JG. Treatment of Parkinson's disease with trophic factors. *Neurotherapeutics.* 2008;5(2):270–280.

35. Braak H, Bohl JR, et al. Stanley Fahn Lecture 2005: The staging procedure for the inclusion body pathology associated with sporadic Parkinson's disease reconsidered. *Mov Disord.* 2006;21(12):2042–2051.

36. Braak H, Muller CM, et al. Pathology associated with sporadic Parkinson's disease—where does it end? *J Neural Transm Suppl.* 2006;(70):89–97.

37. Braak H, Sastre M, et al. Parkinson's disease: lesions in dorsal horn layer I, involvement of parasympathetic and sympathetic pre- and postganglionic neurons. *Acta Neuropathol.* 2007;113(4):421–429.

38. Bjorklund A. Cell therapy for Parkinson's disease: problems and prospects. *Novartis Found Symp.* 2005;265:174–186; discussion 187,204–211.

39. Graff-Radford J, Foote KD, et al. Deep brain stimulation of the internal segment of the globus pallidus in delayed runaway dyskinesia. *Arch Neurol.* 2006;63(8):1181–1184.

40. Linazasoro G. Cell therapy for Parkinson's disease: only young onset patients allowed? Reflections about the results of recent clinical trials with cell therapy and the progression of Parkinson's disease. *Cell Transplant.* 2006;15(6):463–473.

41. Paul G. Cell transplantation for patients with Parkinson's disease. *Handb Exp Pharmacol.* 2006;(174):361–388.

42. Breysse N, Carlsson T, et al. The functional impact of the intrastriatal dopamine neuron grafts in parkinsonian rats is reduced with advancing disease. *J Neurosci.* 2007;27(22):5849–5856.

43. Hall VJ, Li JY, et al. Restorative cell therapy for Parkinson's disease: a quest for the perfect cell. *Semin Cell Dev Biol.* 2007;18(6):859–869.

44. Korecka JA, Verhaagen J, et al. Cell-replacement and gene-therapy strategies for Parkinson's and Alzheimer's disease. *Regen Med.* 2007;2(4):425–446.

45. Polgar S, Ng J. A critical analysis of evidence for using sham surgery in Parkinson's disease: implications for public health. *Aust N Z J Public Health.* 2007;31(3):270–274.

46. Goetz CG, Wuu J, et al. Placebo response in Parkinson's disease: comparisons among 11 trials covering medical and surgical interventions. *Mov Disord.* 2008;23(5):690–699.

47. Stover NP, Watts RL. Spheramine for treatment of Parkinson's disease. *Neurotherapeutics.* 2008;5(2):252–259.

48. Freed CR, Greene PE, et al. Transplantation of embryonic dopamine neurons for severe Parkinson's disease. *N Engl J Med.* 2001;344(10):710–719.

49. Carlsson T, Winkler C, et al. Graft placement and uneven pattern of reinnervation in the striatum is important for development of graft-induced dyskinesia. *Neurobiol Dis.* 2006;21(3):657–668.
50. Olanow CW, Goetz CG, et al. A double-blind controlled trial of bilateral fetal nigral transplantation in Parkinson's disease. *Ann Neurol.* 2003;54(3):403–414.
51. Kordower JH, Chu Y, et al. Lewy body-like pathology in long-term embryonic nigral transplants in Parkinson's disease. *Nat Med.* 2008;14(5):504–506.

I received my very unwelcome Parkinson's disease diagnosis about 2 years ago at age 63. Despite my best efforts and given that 99.97% of the world's population does not seem to have Parkinson's disease, I still suffer badly from the "why me" effect.

I appreciate that there are no magic pills to take the bad feeling away, but what do you tell your patients who find the diagnosis hard to cope with?

As always, many thanks for the time you devote to this forum.

CHAPTER 10

Ten Things on the Horizon for Treating Parkinson's Disease

What are 10 things on the horizon for PD that we can hope for in the next 10 years?

The PD community is lucky because there are thousands of multi/interdisciplinary health care professionals dedicated to research, care, and outreach planet-wide. The network that we have developed is diverse, and so it is difficult to be concrete in making predictions. We hope that there will be more than 10 new and innovative things that will help speed the evolution and fuel the revolution in PD services. For now, we can look forward to the following 10 developments in the field:

1. The development of quality indicators of care in PD that will improve the existence of every PWP on the planet
2. The training of multi/interdisciplinary teams in PD care to enhance the services available to patients
3. Models and criteria for centers of excellence that can be sustainable and opened around the globe
4. New pharmaceutical approaches to PD that will offer disease modification and perhaps even neuroprotection
5. Better medical and surgical treatments for the levodopa-resistant symptoms of speech/swallowing, gait/balance, and cognition
6. Smaller and smarter DBS devices that will be self-contained in the skull and that will be able to sense brain signals and provide automatic symptomatic responses

7. The development of stem cells and viral vectors, and perhaps combinations of the two, for human trials

8. The development of nanotechnological solutions for repairing the brain and for addressing symptomatic problems in PD (a true brain-machine interface)

9. The development of robotic technology and computer-guided assistive devices for PWPs

10. The development of siRNA (small interfering RNA) insertion to interfere with genes and to potentially treat the symptoms of PD

The first three items are already well on their way as focused programs for the NPF, and there are thousands of scientists at work on the final seven. We hope and pray that there will be many more ideas and creative innovations in the years to come, and we believe that there is great hope for the millions of PWPs worldwide.

Appendix

MEDICATIONS USED FOR PARKINSON'S DISEASE

Carbidopa/Levodopa

The primary drug used to relieve PD symptoms is a combination of carbidopa and levodopa. In the brain, levodopa is converted to dopamine, the neurotransmitter that is deficient in PD. Carbidopa allows levodopa to enter the brain with fewer side effects than levodopa alone. The dose is written as a fraction with the top number representing the amount (mg) of carbidopa and the bottom number representing the amount (mg) of levodopa.

Side Effects: As with most medications, side effects may occur when treatment starts, when the dose is changed, or at any time during treatment; not everyone may experience side effects. Potential side effects include nausea, hypotension, dyskinesia, confusion, hallucinations, dystonias, "wearing-off" effect, "on-off" effect, sleepiness, insomnia, dry mouth, skin rash.

Special Considerations: Never abruptly stop carbidopa/levodopa without consulting the health care prescriber. Since carbidopa/levodopa is taken at frequent intervals during the day, patients often use special wristwatches or pillboxes with multiple alarm settings; these are available at many department stores and pharmacies.

Sinemet (carbidopa/levodopa)	Sinemet CR	Parcopa (a form that will dissolve in the mouth)
Available as: 10/100, 25/100, 25/250	Available as: 25/100, 50/200	Available as: 10/100, 25/100, 25/250
Dosing issues: Tablet is s cored (partially cut), so that the tablet may be easily broken in half. Take one-half hour to one hour before meals or two hours after meals. Take with an entire glass of water or juice.	Dosing issues: NEVER chew, crush or cut the controlled-release/ long-acting form (CR). Take with an entire glass of water or juice.	Dosing issues: Can be taken with/without fluid/drink.

Dopamine Agonists

These drugs mimic the effects of dopamine by stimulating dopamine receptors directly. They are most commonly used in combination with carbidopa/levodopa when additional help is needed to control PD symptoms and to smooth out the fluctuations of mobility that occur over time. Dopamine agonists may also be used as initial therapy to delay the need for carbidopa/levodopa.

Side Effects: See individual medication(s).

Special Considerations: Changes in dose (increases and decreases) are made slowly; achieving the best dose may take several weeks. Dizziness, lightheadedness, or headache may indicate medication-related hypotension; evaluate via supine/standing BP measurements over several days. Evaluate/discuss any baseline levels of compulsive behaviors (eg, gambling, hypersexuality) as these behaviors may occur. Potential safety concerns with sudden onset of sleep during activities, including driving, reported with some dopamine agonist use.

Pramipexole dihyrochloride (Mirapex)	Ropinirole (Requip, Requip LA)	Rotigotine (Neupro) Transdermal patch	Bromocriptine mesylate (Parlodel)	Apomorphine (Apokyn)
Available as: .125, .25, .5, 1.0, 1.5mg	*Available as:* .25, .5, 1, 2, 3, 4, 5mg and Long acting 2, 4, 8mg	*Available as:* 2, 4, 6mg patch	*Available as:* 2.5mg tablet 5 mg capsule	Injectable formulation, available in a pen-type injector (SC = under the skin)
Side Effects: Nausea, postural hypotension, hallucinations, constipation, insomnia, somnolence, dyskinesia, dystonia, compulsive behaviors.	*Side Effects:* Nausea, hypotension, somnolence, headache, vomiting, dyskinesia, hallucinations, compulsive behaviors.	*Side Effects:* Skin reactions at patch site, postural hypotension, nausea, vomiting, hallucinations, somnolence, insomnia, applied every 24 hours	*Side Effects:* Postural hypotension, nausea, confusion, hallucinations, dystonia, ergotism, headache,	Primarily used to treat acute "off" periods; requires specific/detailed training. Contraindicated in patients allergic to sulfites or if treated with 5HT3 antagonists such as ondansetron, granisetron, etc.

Please refer to drug reference guides for dose ranges and a complete list of adverse effects.

COMT Inhibitors

These medications block catechol-O-methyltransferase, an enzyme that breaks down dopamine. This action increases the availability of dopamine. COMT inhibitors must be used in combination with carbidopa/levodopa to be effective.

Side Effects: See individual medications.

Special Considerations: Individuals with a history of liver disease should not use these drugs.

Tolcapone (Tasmar)	Carbidopa/levodopa/ entacapone (Stalevo)	Entacapone (Comtan)
Available doses: tablet, 100, 200 mg. *Side effects:* Diarrhea, dyskinesia, hypotension, hallucinations, nausea, urine discoloration. *Special considerations:* The FDA warns that Tasmar should be used as an adjunct only in PWPs on carbidopa/levodopa who are experiencing symptom fluctuation and who are not responding to, or are not appropriate candidates for, other therapies. Tasmar requires liver monitoring due to an increased risk of liver toxicity.	*Available as:* tablets containing # mg cabidopa/# mg levodopa/ # mg entacapone *Available doses:* Stalevo 50: 12.5, 50, 200 mg; Stalevo 100: 25, 100, 200 mg; Stalevo 150: 37.5, 150, 200 mg; Stalevo 200: 50, 200 mg *Side Effects:* Darkened saliva or urine, diarrhea, fatigue, dizziness, abdominal pain, dyskinesia, pain, constipation, hallucinations. *Special considerations:* See carbidopa/levodopa and Comtan (entacapone).	*Available doses:* tablet 200 mg *Side effects:* Diarrhea, dyskinesia, hypotension, hallucinations, nausea, urine discoloration. *Special considerations:* Comtan does not require monitoring of liver function.

MAO Type B Inhibitors

These drugs decrease the breakdown of dopamine. They are used in combination with Sinemet or as a first-time therapy to relieve symptoms of PD.

Side Effects: excessive dopamine symptoms, gastrointestinal upset (insomnia with selegiline).

Special Considerations: Should *not* be taken with Demerol (meperidine). Patients scheduled for elective surgery should notify their health care provider so that the medication is discontinued or appropriate measures are taken. Cautious use with certain SSRIs due to risk of confusion. Last dose should be taken no later than 2:00 PM (risk of insomnia.).

Selegiline 5 mg tablets (Eldepryl)	Orally disintegrating selegiline (Zelapar)	Rasagiline (Azilect tablets 1, 2 mg)
Available as: 5 mg tablets.	Available as: 1.25 mg tablets.	Available as: 0.5 mg and 1.0 mg tablets
	Special considerations: Instruct the patient to let the medication absorb under the tongue. Patient should not eat or drink anything for 5 minutes after medication intake to fully absorb the medication.	Special considerations: A low tyramine diet is recommended; medications such as omeprazole and ciprofloxacin may alter the potency of the medication; try to avoid mixing with cold medications with pseudoephedrine.

Please refer to drug reference guides for dose ranges and a complete list of adverse effects.

Anticholinergics

These drugs are primarily used to treat tremor early in the course of treatment. They help maintain a proper balance of brain chemicals acetylcholine and dopamine.

Side Effects: Dry mouth, blurred vision, urinary retention, confusion, hallucinations, sedation, constipation, vomiting, loss of appetite, weight loss, listlessness, nervousness.

Special Considerations: Persons with glaucoma should not use this medication. The side effects of confusion or difficulty urinating may necessitate halting the use of this medication.

Amantadine* (Symmetrel)	Benztropine mesylate (Cogentin)	Biperiden hydrochloride (Akineton)	Procyclidine hydrochloride (Kemadrin)	Trihexyphenidyl HCL (Artane)
Available doses: Capsules 100 mg, liquid syrup *Side effects:* Swelling of ankles and legs, "livido reticularis," hallucinations, confusion *Special considerations:* Amantadine should be used cautiously in patients who have heart and/or renal failure.	*Available doses:* tablets 0.5 mg, 1.0 mg, 2.0 mg	*Available doses:* tablets 2 mg	*Available doses:* tablets 5 mg	*Available doses:* tablets 2, 5 mg

*Amantadine is an antiviral compound believed to boost the release of dopamine in the brain.

Please refer to drug reference guides for dose ranges and a complete list of adverse effects.

Source: Adapted from Tuite PJ, Thomas CA, Reukert LF, Fernandez HH. *Parkinson's Disease: A Guide to Patient Care*, New York, NY: Springer Publishing Company; 2009: 275–279.

MEDICATION SCHEDULE

Photocopy and complete this form and bring it with you to your clinic visits.

Name _____   Effective Date: _____ / _____ / _____

Neurologist _____   Contact Info: _____

Primary Care _____   Contact Info: _____

Pharmacy _____   Contact Info: _____

Medications	Dose	Times										
Additional instructions:												

PARKINSON'S DISEASE SYMPTOMS

Photocopy and mark the symptoms that pertain to you for discussion with your doctor.

Common Problems in Parkinsonism and/or Side Effects of Medication

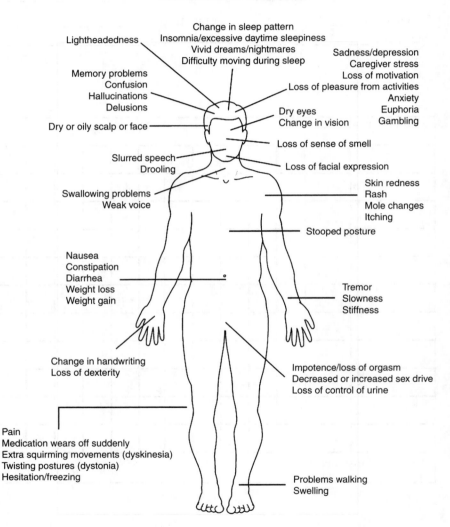

"The Parkinson's Person," courtesy of Dr. Kimberly Trinidad and Patricia Weigel from the University at Buffalo Movement Disorders Center.

Resources

LAY NATIONAL ORGANIZATIONS

National Parkinson Foundation
www.parkinson.org
1501 NW 9th Avenue/Bob Hope Rd
Miami, FL 33136-1494
Telephone: 305-243-6666
Toll-free: 1-800-327-4545
Fax: 305-243-5595
E-mail: contact@parkinson.org

Discussion Forums:
Ask the Doctor; Ask the Surgical Team; Ask About Nutrition;
Ask the Spanish Doctor; Talk to a Speech Clinician
http://forum.parkinson.org/forum/

American Parkinson Disease Association (APDA)
www.apdaparkinson.org
135 Parkinson Avenue
Staten Island, NY 10305
Telephone: 1-800-223-2732 or 718-981-8001
Fax: 718-981-4399
E-mail: apda@apdaparkinson.org

APDA National Young Onset Center
Glenbrook Hospital
2100 Pfingsten Rd

Glenview Hospital
Glenview, IL 60026
Telephone: 877-223-3801
Fax: 847-657-5708
E-mail: apda@youngparkinson.org

European Parkinson's Disease Association
www.epda.eu.com
Telephone/Fax: +44 (0) 1732-457-683

Hong Kong Parkinson's Disease Foundation
www.hkpdf.org.hk/

Michael J. Fox Foundation for Parkinson's Research
www.MichaelJFox.org
The Michael J. Fox Foundation for Parkinson's Research
Church Street Station
PO Box 780
New York, NY 10008-0780
Telephone: 1-800-708-7644

Malaysian Parkinson's Disease Association
http://www.mpda.org.my
35 Jalan Nyaman 10, Happy Garden,
58200 Kuala Lumpur
Telephone: 03-7980-6685
Fax: 03-7982-6685

Parkinson's Disease Foundation
www.pdf.org
1359 Broadway, Suite 1509
New York, NY 10018
Telephone: 1-800-457-6676 or 212-923-4700
Fax: 212-923-4778
E-mail: info@pdf.org

Parkinson's Disease Foundation of India
www.parkinsonsdiseaseindia.com
302, Jaltarang, Kishore Kumar Lane
Juhu Tara Rd, Mumbai 400 049
Telephone: 26604525 or 26607845

Parkinson's Action Network
www.parkinsonsaction.org
Parkinson's Action Network
1025 Vermont Ave NW Suite 1120
Washington, DC 20005
Telephone: 202-638-4101
Toll-free: 1-800-850-4726
Fax: 202-638-7257
E-mail: info@parkinsonsaction.org

Parkinson Alliance
www.parkinsonalliance.org
The Parkinson Alliance
PO Box 308
Kingston, NJ 08528-0308
Telephone: 1-800-579-8440 or 609-688-0870
Fax: 609-688-0875

Parkinson Society Canada
http://www.parkinson.ca
4211 Yonge St, 316 Toronto, ON M2P 2A9
Telephone: 416-227-9700
Fax: 416-227-9600
Toll-free: 1-800-565-3000

Parkinson's Western Australia
www.parkinsonswa.org.au
Centre for Neurological Support
The Niche Suite B,
11 Aberdare Rd
Nedlands, WA 6009
Telephone: 08-9346-7373
Fax: 08-9346-7374

WE MOVE Worldwide Education and Awareness for Movement Disorders
www.wemove.org 204 W 84th St New York, NY 10024
E-mail: wemove@wemove.org

World Parkinson Disease Association
http://www.wpda.org/

World Parkinson Congress
www.worldpdcongress.org

PROFESSIONAL ORGANIZATIONS

American Academy of Neurology (AAN)
www.aan.com
1080 Montreal Avenue
Saint Paul, MN 55116
Telephone: 1-800-879-1960 or 651-695-2717
Fax: 651-695-2791
E-mail: memberservices@aan.com

American Association of Neuroscience Nurses
www.aann.org
4700 W Lake Avenue
Glenview, IL 60025
Telephone: 888-557-2266 (US only) or 847-375-4733
Fax: 847-375-6430
International Fax: 732-460-7313
E-mail: info@aann.org

American Medical Directors Association
www.amda.com
11000 Broken Land Parkway, Suite 400
Columbia, MD 21044
Telephone: 410-740-9743
Toll-free: 1-800-876-2632
Fax: 410-740-4572

American Physical Therapy Association
www.apta.org
1111 N Fairfax St
Alexandria, VA 22314-1488
Telephone: 1-800-999-APTA (2782) or 703-684-APTA (2782)
Fax: 703-684-7343

American Occupational Therapy Association
www.aota.org
4720 Montgomery Lane
PO Box 31220
Bethesda, MD 20824-1220
Telephone: 301-652-2682
Toll-free: 1-800-377-8555
Fax: 301-652-7711

American Speech-Language-Hearing Association
www.asha.org
ASHA National Office
2200 Research Boulevard
Rockville, MD 20850-3289
Telephone: 301-296-5700

Movement Disorder Society
www.movementdisorders.org
International Secretariat
555 E Wells St, Suite 1100
Milwaukee, WI 53202-3823
Telephone: +1 414-276-2145
Fax: +1 414-276-3349
E-mail: info@movementdisorders.org

National Association of Social Workers
www.socialworkers.org
750 First St, NE, Suite 700
Washington, DC 20002-4241
Telephone: 202-408-8600

INFORMATION ON PARKINSON'S DISEASE RESEARCH STUDIES AND CLINICAL TRIALS

PD Trials
www.pdtrials.org
Telephone: 1-800-457-6676
E-mail: info@pdtrials.org

An initiative to increase education and awareness of clinical trials led by the Parkinson's Disease Foundation in collaboration with other organizations.

Parkinson Study Group
www.parkinson-study-group.org
University of Rochester
1351 Mt Hope Avenue, Suite 223
Rochester, NY 14620

A cooperative group of Parkinson's disease experts from medical centers in the United States and Canada who are dedicated to improving treatment for persons affected by Parkinson's disease.

National Institutes of Health
www.clinical trials.gov

National Institute of Neurological Disorders and Stroke
www.ninds.nih.gov

Parkinson's Disease Pipeline
www.pdpipeline.org

Further Reading

Bunting LK, Vernon GM. *Comprehensive Nursing Care for Parkinson's Disease.* New York, NY: Springer; 2007.

Calne SM, Kumar A. Nursing care of patients with late-stage Parkinson's disease. *J Neurosci Nurs.* 2003;35:242–251.

Carter JH, Stewart BJ, Archbold, et al. Living with a person who has Parkinson's disease: the spouse's perspective by stage of disease. *Mov Disord.* 1998;13:20–28.

Chou KL, Evatt M, Hinson V, Kompoliti K. Sialorrhea in Parkinson's disease: a review. *Mov Disord.* 2007;22:2306–2313.

Ellis T, Katz DI, White DK, DePiero TJ, Hohler AD, Saint-Hilaire MH. Effectiveness of an inpatient multidisciplinary rehabilitation program for patients with Parkinson's disease. *Physical Therapy.* 2008;88(7):1–8.

Emre M, Aarsland D, Albanese A, et al. Rivastigmine for dementia associated with Parkinson's disease. *N Engl J Med.* 2004;351:2509–2518.

Evans AH, Katzenschlager R, Paviour D, et al. Punding in Parkinson's disease: its relation to the dopamine dysregulation syndrome. *Mov Disord.* 2004;19:397–405.

Fernandez HH, Friedman JH. Punding on L-Dopa. *Mov Disord.* 1999;14:836–838.

Friedman JH. *Making the Connection Between Brain and Behavior-Coping with Parkinson's Disease.* New York, NY: Demos Health; 2008.

Friedman JH, Fernandez HH. Non-motor problems in Parkinson's disease. *Neurolog.* 2000;6(1):18–27.

Hanagasi HA, Emre M. Treatment of behavioural symptoms and dementia in Parkinson's disease. *Fundam Clin Pharmacol.* 2005;19:133–146.

Holden K. *Parkinson's Disease: Guidelines for Medical Nutrition Therapy.* Five Star Living, Inc; 2000.

Keus SHJ, Bloem B, Hendriks EJ, Bredero-Cohen AB, Munneke M; Practice Recommendations Development Group. Evidence-based analysis of physical therapy in Parkinson's disease with recommendations for practice and research. *Mov Disord.* 2007;22(4):451–460

Loew JE, Pratt C. *Good Nutrition and Parkinson's Disease.* American Parkinson's Disease Association, Inc; 2007.

Lyons KS, Stewart BJ, Archbold PG, Carter JH, Perrin NA. Pessimism & optimism as early warning signs for health decline in Parkinson's disease caregivers. *Nurs Res.* 2004;53:354–362.

Marjama-Lyons JM, Koller WC. Parkinson's disease: update in diagnosis and symptom management. *Geriatrics.* 2001;56:24–35.

Meyer MM, Derr P, Imke S. *The Comfort of Home for Parkinson's Disease: A Guide for Caregivers.* Portland, OR: Care Trust; 2007.

Miyasaki JM, Martin W, Suchowersky O, et al. Practice parameter: initiation of treatment for Parkinson's disease: an evidence-based review. Report of the quality standards subcommittee of the American Academy of Neurology. *Neurology.* 2002;58:11–17.

Muller T. Drug treatment of non-motor symptoms in Parkinson's disease. *Expert Opin Pharmacother.* 2002;3:381–388.

Okun MS, Fernandez HH, Rodriguez RL, Foote KD. Identifying candidates for deep brain stimulation in Parkinson's disease: the role of the primary care physician. *Geriatrics.* 2007;62(5):18–24.

Okun MS, Rodriguez RL, Foote KD, et al. A case-based review of troubleshooting deep brain stimulator issues in movement and neuropsychiatric disorders. *Parkinsonism Relat Disord.* 2008;14(7):532–538.

Rabinstein AA, Shulman LM. Management of behavioral and psychiatric problems in Parkinson's disease. *Parkinsonism Relat Disord.* 2000;7:41–50.

Ravina B, Putt M, Siderowf A, et al. Donepezil for dementia in Parkinson's disease: a randomized, double-blind, placebo-controlled, crossover study. *J Neurol Neurosurg Psychiatry.* 2005;76(7):934–939.

Rodriguez RL, Fernandez HH, Haq I, Okun MS. Pearls in patient selection for deep brain stimulation. *Neurologist.* Sep 2007;13(5):253–260.

Shapiro MA, Chang YL, Munson SK, et al. 4 "A"s associated with pathological Parkinson gamblers: anxiety, anger, age and agonists. *Neuropsychiatr Dis Treat.* 2007;3(2):1–7.

Uc EY, Struck LK, Rodnitzky RL et al. Predictors of weight loss in Parkinson's disease. *Mov Disord.* 2006;21(7):930–936.

Voon V, Hassan K, Zurowski M, et al. Prevalence of repetitive and reward-seeking behaviors in Parkinson disease. *Neurology.* 2006;67:1254–1257.

Waters CH. Treatment of advanced stage patients with Parkinson's disease. *Parkinsonism Relat Disord.* 2002;9:15–21.

Zahodne LB, Fernandez HH. Course prognosis and management of psychosis in Parkinson's disease: are current treatments really effective? *CNS Spectr.* 2008;13(3)(Suppl 4):26–34.

Zahodne, L, Fernandez HH. Pathophysiology and treatment of psychosis in Parkinson's disease: a review. *Drugs and Aging* 2008;25(8):665–682.

About the Authors

Michael S. Okun, MD, received his BA in History from Florida State University and his MD from the University of Florida where he graduated with honors. Dr. Okun completed an internship and neurology residency at the University of Florida. Following residency he was trained at Emory University, one of the world's leading centers for movement disorders research, in both general movement disorders and in microelectrode recording/surgical treatments. He is currently codirector of the Movement Disorders Center located within the McKnight Brain Institute and the University of Florida College of Medicine. The center is unique in that it comprises more than 25 interdisciplinary faculty members from diverse areas of campus, all of whom are dedicated to care, outreach, education, and research. Dr. Okun has been dedicated to this interdisciplinary care concept, and since his appointment as the national medical director for the National Parkinson Foundation (NPF) in 2006, he has worked with the 59 NPF centers to help foster the best possible environments for care, research, and outreach in Parkinson's disease. Dr. Okun has been supported by grants from the NPF, the National Institutes of Health, the Parkinson Alliance, and the Michael J. Fox Foundation for Parkinson's Disease Research, and he currently administers the online international "ask the expert forums," on the NPF website. Dr. Okun has not only dedicated much of his career to helping in the development of care centers for people suffering with movement disorders but has also has enjoyed a prolific research career exploring nonmotor basal ganglia brain features, and he has participated in some of the pioneering studies exploring the cognitive, behavioral, and mood effects of brain stimulation. Dr. Okun is one of the most published authors in the area of surgical intervention for Parkinson's disease (PD) and movement disorders. Dr. Okun holds the Adelaide Lackner Associate Professorship in Neurology, has published over 100 peer-reviewed articles, is a published poet (*Lessons From the Bedside*, 1995), and has served as a reviewer for more than 25 major medical journals. He has been invited to speak about PD and movement disorders in various regions throughout the world, and he is currently a faculty and founding member for SUPPORT-PD, which aims to bring functional Parkinson's and movement disorders surgery to "countries in need" around the globe. Dr. Okun is also a loving husband to Leslie Smith Okun (a violinist and nurse) and a wonderful father to two-year-old Jack Robert Okun. Leslie and Michael are expecting their second child at the time of publication of this book.

Hubert H. Fernandez, MD, is associate professor of Neurology, director of Clinical Trials for Movement Disorders, codirector of the Movement Disorders Program, and Associate Chair of Academic Affairs, Department of Neurology, all at the University of Florida. He is also the medical director of the University of Florida's NPF Center of Excellence and Tyler's Hope Center for Comprehensive Dystonia Care. He received his medical degree in the Philippines and completed his neurology residency at Boston University and a postgraduate fellowship in movement disorders at Brown University.

Dr. Fernandez is a Fellow of the American Academy of Neurology (also executive board member of its movement disorders section) and an active member of several professional societies, including the American Neurological Association, The Movement Disorder Society (also a member of the Scientific Issues Committee and chair of the Task Force on Psychosis Scales), and the Florida Society of Neurology (also an executive board member and the president-elect). He is an active participant of several consortiums of academic clinical trial investigators such as the Parkinson Study Group (also cochair of the Functional Neurosurgical Working Group), Dystonia Study Group (also a member of the executive board), and the Huntington Study Group. Dr. Fernandez has been the lead or senior author of five other books (*Ultimate Review for the Neurology Boards*, Demos Publishing; *The Practical Approach to Any Movement Disorder*, Demos Publishing; *Clinician's Desk Reference: Parkinson's Disease*, Manson Publishing Ltd; *Parkinson's Disease: A Guide to Patient Care*, Springer Publishing; *Ultimate Review for the Neurology Boards, Expanded 2nd Edition*, Demos Publishing), over two dozen book chapters, and over 150 scientific abstracts. He has authored over 150 peer-reviewed clinical publications on PD and other movement disorders, in the area of clinical trials, long-term care, and drug therapy; he is one of the world's leading experts in the area of nonmotor aspects of PD, especially behavioral and cognitive dysfunction. He is currently serving on the editorial board of *Movement Disorders* and *Clinical Neuropharmacology*, and is an ad hoc reviewer for more than a dozen peer-reviewed journals, including *New England Journal of Medicine, Neurology, Annals of Neurology, Parkinsonism and Related Disorders, Journal of Neurology, Neurosurgery and Psychiatry, Journal of Clinical Psychiatry,* and *European Journal of Neurology.* Dr. Fernandez has initiated or participated in over three dozen single-center and multicenter clinical trials and has served as the national principal investigator for the United States in several global studies. He currently serves as the medical editor of the Movement Disorder Society website (www.movementdisorders.org). He is the father of a beautiful 10-year-old, Annella Marie Fernandez, and husband to a fellow clinician-researcher-educator, Maria Cecilia Lansang, who is also the current interim chief of the Division of Endocrinology at the University of Florida.

Index

AAC treatment. *See* Augmentative-
    alternative communication
    (AAC) treatment
AAV. *See* Adeno-associated virus
    (AAV)
Acupuncture, 132–133
AD. *See* Alzheimer's disease (AD)
Adeno-associated virus (AAV), 194
Alpha-synuclein protein, 14
Alternative or complementary
    medications, used in
    Parkinson's disease
  acupuncture, 132–133
  chelation therapy, 138
  coenzyme Q10, 135
  creatine, 135–136
  dehydroepiandrosterone, 137–138
  glutathione, 136–137
  hair analysis, 138
  herbal remedies, 131
  massage therapy, 133
  Mucuna pruriens, 132
  tai chi, 133
  vitamin E, 136
Alzheimer's disease (AD), 14
  difference with Parkinson's
      disease, 20
  symptomatic treatments for, 20

Amantadine, 100
Amphetamine metabolites, 102
Anticholinergic drugs, 21, 100–101,
    212
Antidepressants, in treating depres-
    sion in Parkinson's disease, 113
  side effects of, 114
Anxiety, 84–85
Apathy, 83–84
Apomorphine, 111–112
Atherosclerotic disease, 81
Auditory hallucinations, 85. *See also*
    Visual hallucinations
Augmentative-alternative communi-
    cation (AAC) treatment, 138
Autonomic dysfunction, treatments of,
    119–120

Basal ganglia, 153
Beck depression inventory-I
    (BDI-I), 22
Behavioral complications, in
    Parkinson's disease, 82
Benefits of exercise, in treatment of
    PD, 134
Best Medical Therapy (BMT), 176
Biomarkers, for Parkinson's disease, 3
Bladder hyperactivity, 80

Bladder outlet obstruction, 81
Blood-brain barrier, 21, 22, 108
Blood markers, 3
Blood test, to diagnose Parkinson's
    disease, 6
BMT. See Best Medical Therapy (BMT)
Bradykinesia, implication in
    Parkinson's disease, 62, 107
Brain cells, 3, 7
Brain degeneration, 12
Brain lesions, pressure effects of, 19
Bromocriptine, 105

Cancer treatment, for PWP, 53
Carbidopa, 108
    different forms of, 108–110
Catechol-O-methyltransferase
    (COMT) inhibitors, 111
CBD. See Corticobasal degeneration
    (CBD)
CDNF. See Conserved dopamine
    neurotropic factor (CDNF)
Cell-based therapy, 197
Chelation therapy, for treating
    Parkinson's disease, 138
Cholinesterase inhibitors, 115
Coenzyme Q10, 135
Cognitive behavioral therapy, 83
Cognitive dysfunction, 15
Cogwheel rigidity, 63
Compulsive eating, 89
Compulsive medication use, 90
Compulsive shopping, 88–89
COMT inhibitors. See Catechol-O-
    methyltransferase (COMT)
    inhibitors
Conserved dopamine neurotropic
    factor (CDNF), 195
Constipation, 141
Corticobasal degeneration (CBD), 13,
    174
    symptoms for, 16
    treatment of, 16
Creatine dietary supplement, 135–136

DATATOP. See Deprenyl and
    Tocopherol Antioxidative
    Therapy of Parkinsonism
    (DATATOP)
Deep brain stimulation (DBS), 19,
    29–30, 65, 167
    assessment for cognitive
        dysfunction for, 177
    availability of, 184
    commitment required by patients
        registered for, 173
    complications of, 177–181
    electric shock-like sensations
        during, 181
    laws governing use of, 183
    patient selection procedure for,
        172–173
    side effects encountered with, 182
    symptoms of Parkinson's disease
        responsive to, 174
'Deep tissue' massage, 133
Dehydration, in PD patient, 47
Dehydroepiandrosterone (DHEA),
    137–138
Delusions, 85
Deprenyl and Tocopherol
    Antioxidative Therapy of
    Parkinsonism (DATATOP), 102
Depression, 4, 82
    difference with apathy, 83–84
    drugs for treatment of, 113–115
DHEA. See Dehydroepiandrosterone
    (DHEA)
Diagnostic markers, for Parkinson's
    disease, 4
Dietary supplements, in Parkinson's
    disease, 134–135
Disorders and syndromes, hav-
    ing symptoms similar to
    Parkinson's disease, 12–13
Doctors treating Parkinson's disease,
    training requirements for, 6–7
Dopamine agonists, 105–106
Dopamine decarboxylase, 21

Dopaminergic cells, 65
Dopaminergic medications, 14, 83
Dopaminergic neurons, 4
Dopaminergic therapy, 50
Dose failure, 69
Drugs, for improving concentration and memory in Parkinson's disease, 115–116
Dyskinesias, 66–67, 70, 100
Dystonia, 68

Earlier vs Later L-DOPA (ELLDOPA), 107
ECG. *See* Electrocardiogram (ECG)
ECT. *See* Electroconvulsive therapy (ECT)
EECP. *See* Enhanced external counter-pulsation (EECP)
EEG. *See* Electroencephalogram (EEG)
Electrocardiogram (ECG), 30
Electroconvulsive therapy (ECT), 83
Electroencephalogram (EEG), 30
ELLDOPA. *See* Earlier vs Later L-DOPA (ELLDOPA)
EMST. *See* Expiratory muscle strength training (EMST)
Enhanced external counterpulsation (EECP), 137
Entacapone, 108
Erectile dysfunction, 45–46, 120
Essential tremor (ET)
  difference with PD, 18–19
  treatments for, 19
Experimental animal model, of PD, 10
Expiratory muscle strength training (EMST), 139

Freezing, motor fluctuation, 69–70

GAD. *See* Glutamic acid decarboxylase (GAD)
Gamma knife radiosurgery, for treatment of Parkinson's disease, 184
Gastroparesis, 141

GDNF. *See* Glial cell-derived neurotrophic factor (GDNF)
Gene tests, for diagnosis of Parkinson's disease, 8
Gene therapy, 193–194
  trials for Parkinson's disease, 194–195
Glial cell-derived neurotrophic factor (GDNF), 194, 195
Globus pallidus interna (GPi), 177
Glutamic acid decarboxylase (GAD), 194
Glutathione, use in treatment of Parkinson's disease, 136–137
GPi. *See* Globus pallidus interna (GPi)

Hair analysis, 138
Hallucinations, 14. *See also* Auditory hallucinations; Visual hallucinations
Health Information Privacy Act (HIPPA), 45
Hemi-body parkinsonism, 62
Hemi-parkinsonism syndrome, 62
Herbal remedies, for treatment for Parkinson's disease, 131
HIPPA. *See* Health Information Privacy Act (HIPPA)
Hospitalization, need in case of PD, 25
Huntington's disease, 8
Hypersexuality, 46, 88
Hypokinesia, 62
Hypophonia, 62

Impaired reality testing, 86
Impulse control disorder (ICD), 87
  process for treatment of, 117–118
Insomnia, 75, 113
Intracranial lesions, 19

Lead-pipe rigidity, 63
Lee Silverman Voice Therapy (LSVT), 138–139
Lesion therapy, 19

Levodopa therapy, 90, 107
    different forms of, 108–110
    effect of disease progression
        during, 67
    and effect on progression of
        Parkinson's disease, 110
    medications avoided in combination
        with, 122
    motor complications of, 66
    for Parkinson's disease, 5–6
    side effects of, 207
Lewy body disease, 13, 174
    treatment for, 14–15
LSVT. See Lee Silverman Voice
    Therapy (LSVT)
Lumbar disc disease, 51
Lumbosacral spine, 51

Macrostimulation, 170
Magnetic resonance angiography
    (MRA), 19
MAOB inhibitors, 101
MAOIs. See Monoamine oxidase
    inhibitors (MAOIs)
Massage therapy, for treating PD, 133
Medications
    avoided during Parkinson's
        disease, 121
    used for treating Parkinson's
        disease, 26–27
        anticholinergics, 212
        carbidopa/levodopa, 207–208
        COMT inhibitors, 210
        dopamine agonists, 208–209
        MAO type B inhibitors, 211
    used to treat psychosis in
        Parkinson's disease, 116–117
Memantine drug, for treatment
    of dementia in Parkinson's
    disease, 115
Microcarrier support matrix, 197
Microelectrodes, 169–171
Micrographia, 62
Monoamine oxidase inhibitors
    (MAOIs), 29, 83

Motor complications, in Parkinson's
    disease, 65–66
Motor symptoms, for Parkinson's
    disease, 61
Movement disorders, 51
Movement disorders neurologist, role
    of, 152
MRA. See Magnetic resonance
    angiography (MRA)
Mucuna pruriens, 132
Multi- and interdisciplinary approach,
    in treatment of PD, 151
Multiple system atrophy (MSA), 13,
    174
    symptoms of, 15

Neurodegenerative disorder, 7
Nonmotor symptoms, of Parkinson's
    disease, 75
Normal pressure hydrocephalus
    (NPH), 24–25
Nutritionist, role of, 156–157

Obsessive-compulsive disorder (OCD),
    89–90
Obstructive sleep apnea, 48
Occupational risks, for development of
    Parkinson's disease, 44–45
Occupational therapist, role of,
    154–155
OCD. See Obsessive-compulsive
    disorder (OCD)
On-off fluctuations, 69
Opamine-replacement therapy, 66
Orthostasis, 15
Orthostatic hypotension, 80, 120
Osteoporosis, 52–53

Palliative therapy, for treatment of
    Parkinson's disease, 159
Paralysis agitans, 5
Parkinsonian tremor, 64
Parkinsonism, 13
Parkinson motor scores, 106
Parkinson-plus syndrome, 13, 80

Parkinson's disease (PD). *See also*
  Person with Parkinson's (PWP)
  disease
alternative or complementary
  medications used in
  acupuncture, 132–133
  chelation therapy, 138
  coenzyme Q10, 135
  creatine, 135–136
  dehydroepiandrosterone,
    137–138
  glutathione, 136–137
  hair analysis, 138
  herbal remedies, 131
  massage therapy, 133
  Mucuna pruriens, 132
  tai chi, 133
  vitamin E, 136
antidepressants in treating
  depression in, 113
  side effects of, 114
behavioral complications in, 82
benefits of exercise in, 134
biomarker for, 3
blood test for diagnosing, 6
bradykinesia and its implication
  in, 62
cancer treatment and, 53
causes of sleep disturbances in,
  75–77
depression in, 82–83
development of levodopa as therapy
  for, 5–6
diagnostic markers for, 4
dietary supplements safe in,
  134–135
difference between multi-and
  interdisciplinary approach
  in treatment of, 151
difference with
  Alzheimer's disease, 20
  essential tremor, 18–19
disorders and syndromes having
  symptoms similar to, 12–13

drugs for improving concentration
  and memory in, 115–116
effect of stress on, 52
experimental animal model of, 10
gamma knife radiosurgery for, 184
gene therapy trials for, 194–195
history of, 5
hospitalization, 25
impact on work performance due
  to, 43
inappropriate laughing and crying
  in, 22
innovative things revolutionizing
  services associated with,
  205–206
intrinsic and iatrogenic nonmotor
  features in, 76
laws about informing employer
  about, 45
main theories for cause of, 24
medications avoided during, 121
medications used for, 26–27
  anticholinergics, 212
  carbidopa/levodopa, 207–208
  COMT inhibitors, 210
  dopamine agonists, 208–209
  MAO type B inhibitors, 211
medications used to treat psychosis
  in, 116–117
motor complications in, 65–66
motor symptoms in, 61
nonmotor symptoms for (*See*
  Nonmotor symptoms, for
  Parkinson's disease)
nonpharmacological approaches to
  sleep disturbances in, 142
nonpharmacologic remedies for
  autonomic disturbances in, 143
occupational risks for development
  of, 44–45
occurrence of first symptom for, 4–5
parts of brain degenerating in,
  23–24
pathological gambling in, 87–88

Parkinson's disease (PD). (*continued*)
  patients. (*See also* Person with
      Parkinson's (PWP) disease)
    affect on sex life, 45–46
    behavioral complications in, 82
    capacity to make financial
        decisions, 49–50
    communication with children,
        51–52
    daytime sleepiness, 79
    driving car or operating airplane,
        50
    employment status, 43
    flying in airplanes, 47–48
    global positioning system (GPS)
        devices, 47
    going on vacation, 46–47
    medication regimen in case of
        flying overseas, 48
    minimum hours required for
        sleeping, 48
    participation in sports, 48–49
    risks of side-effects of shingles/
        pneumovax vaccine, 53
  persons expected to suffer from, 10
  PET or SPECT scan for diagnosis of,
      11–12
  precautions for
    driving car or operating airplane,
        50
    flying in airplanes, 47–48
    participation in sports, 48–49
    patients going on vacation,
        46–47
    visiting high altitude places,
        47–48
  problems/challenges of stem cells
      for, 192
  psychosis in, 85–86
  results of transplant trials for,
      195–196
  rigidity in, 63
  risk factor for development of, 8–10
  role in treatment of movement
      disorders neurologist, 152
    nutritionist, 156–157
    occupational therapist, 154–155
    physical therapist, 154
    psychiatrist, 153
    social worker, 155–156
    speech therapist, 156–157
  screening tests for, 3
  symptomatic drug therapy in, 97
  symptoms for, 3–4
  symptoms of autonomic dysfunction
      in, 79–81
  timeline for stem cell breakthroughs
      in, 193
  training necessary for doctors
      treating, 6–7
  treatment of
    alternative or complementary
        medications used in, 131–138
    autonomic dysfunction in PD,
        119–120
    difficult-to-control tremor
        associated with PD, 20–21
    exercise or tandem biking
        for, 49
    palliative therapy for, 158
    surgical approaches to, 167
    therapies used for, 99
    use of vitamin E in, 136
  tremors specific to, 63
  use of exercise or tandem biking for
      treating, 49
Parkinson's Rasagiline: Efficacy and
    Safety in the Treatment of OFF
    (PRESTO), 103
Pathological gambling, 87–88
PD. *See* Parkinson's disease (PD)
Periodic leg movements of sleep
    (PMLS), 77
Person with Parkinson's (PWP)
    disease, 4, 24, 28
  affect on sex life of, 45–46
  assistive devices and 'home
      remedies' for, 139–140
  behavioral complications in, 82
  bladder hyperactivity in, 80

cancer treatment for, 53
capacity to make financial decisions by, 49–50
communication with children by, 51–52
compulsive eating among, 89
compulsive shopping among, 88–89
daytime sleepiness, 79
development of psychosis in, 85–86
driving car or operating airplane by, 50
employment status of, 43
flying in airplanes by, 47–48
global positioning system (GPS) devices for, 47
going on vacation, 46–47
hypersexuality among, 46, 88
medication regimen in case of flying overseas, 48
minimum hours required for sleeping, 48
objectives of managing, 110
Parkinson's 'support group' for, 145
participation in sports, 48–49
postural instability in, 64
potential risks associated with pregnancy for, 52
precautions for
    driving car or operating airplane, 50
    flying in airplanes, 47–48
    participation in sports, 48–49
    patients going on vacation, 46–47
    visiting high altitude places, 47–48
risks of side-effects of shingles/pneumovax vaccine on, 53
sleep disorders in, 75
techniques for improving writing difficulties in, 140
types of psychological support available for, 141

visiting high altitude places, 47–48
PET. See Positron emission tomography (PET)
Physical therapist, role of, 154
PMLS. See Periodic leg movements of sleep (PMLS)
Positron emission tomography (PET), 6
Postural instability, 64
Pramipexole, 105
Precautions, for person suffering from PD
    driving car or operating airplane, 50
    flying in airplanes, 47–48
    participation in sports, 48–49
    patients going on vacation, 46–47
    visiting high altitude places, 47–48
PRESTO. See Parkinson's Rasagiline: Efficacy and Safety in the Treatment of OFF (PRESTO)
Progressive Supranuclear Palsy (PSP), 64, 174
    pathology of, 17
    treatment for, 16–17
Psychiatrist, role of, 153
Psychosis, in Parkinson's disease, 85–86
    medications used for treating, 116–117
Psychotherapy, 83
Punding, 89
PWP. See Person with Parkinson's (PWP) disease

Radiosurgery, benefits of, 184
Rapid eye movement (REM), 4, 48, 78–79
Rasagiline, 102–103
Repetitive transcranial magnetic stimulation, 83
Restless legs syndrome (RLS), 77
    treatment for, 118–119
Rigidity, implication in Parkinson's disease, 63

Risk factor, for development of Parkinson's disease, 8–10
RLS. *See* Restless legs syndrome (RLS)
Rotigotine patch, 106

Screening tests, for Parkinson's disease, 3
Selegiline, 102
Serotonin norepinephrine reuptake inhibitors (SNRIs), 83
Serotonin syndrome, 104
Serotonin toxicity, 105
Sexual dysfunction, 45–46
Sinemet, 108
Sinemet-induced nausea, 21
Single photon emission computed tomography (SPECT), 6
Sleep disorders, 4, 48
    causes in Parkinson's disease, 75–77
    as nonmotor problem in Parkinson's disease, 75
    nonpharmacological approaches to sleep disturbances in, 142
    pharmacological treatment of, 119
SLP. *See* Speech-language pathologist (SLP)
SNRIs. *See* Serotonin norepinephrine reuptake inhibitors (SNRIs)
Social worker, role of, 155–156
SPECT. *See* Single photon emission computed tomography (SPECT)
Speech-language pathologist (SLP), 140
Speech therapist, role of, 156–157
Spheramine, cell-based therapy, 197
STalevo Reduction in Dyskinesia Evaluation (STRIDE), 108
Start hesitation, 69
Stem cells, 191–192
    affect of changes in political administration on research of, 193
    application as potential savior therapy for, 192

timeline for breakthroughs in treating PD, 193
transplant, 198
STN. *See* Subthalamic nucleus (STN)
STRIDE. *See* STalevo Reduction in Dyskinesia Evaluation (STRIDE)
Substantia nigra, 3
Subthalamic nucleus (STN), 177
Symptomatic drug therapy, in PD, 97
Symptoms, for PD, 3–4

Tacrine inhibitors, 115
Tai chi, for treatment of Parkinson's disease, 133
Tau protein, 14
TCA. *See* Tricyclic antidepressants (TCA)
TEMPO trial, 103
Tourette's syndrome, 167
Transplant trials, results in case of PD, 195–196
Treatment of Parkinson's disease
    alternative or complementary medications used in, 131–138
    autonomic dysfunction in, 119–120
    difficult-to-control tremor associated with, 20–21
    exercise or tandem biking for, 49
    palliative therapy for, 158
    surgical approaches to, 167
    therapies used for, 99
    use of vitamin E in, 136
Tremors, specific to PD, 63
Tricyclic antidepressants (TCA), 83
TVP-1012 in early monotherapy for PD outpatients. *See* TEMPO trial

Unified Parkinson's Disease Rating Scale (UPDRS), 112, 175, 194

VAMS. *See* Visual analog mood scale (VAMS)
Vascular parkinsonism, 13, 174
    symptoms for, 17

treatment for, 17–18
Visual analog mood scale (VAMS), 22
Visual hallucinations, 85. *See also*
    Auditory hallucinations
Vitamin E, role in treatment of
    Parkinson's disease, 136

Wearing off, 67–68

Yawning, link with dopamine,
    10–11

Zydis selegiline, 105